Sociology and Health Care

AN INTRODUCTION FOR NURSES, MIDWIVES AND ALLIED HEALTH PROFESSIONALS

Michael Sheaff

Open University Press

Open University Press
McGraw-Hill Education
McGraw-Hill House
Shoppenhangers Road
Maidenhead
Berkshire
England
SL6 2QL

email: enquiries@openup.co.uk
world wide web: www.openup.co.uk
and Two Penn Plaza, New York, NY 10121-2289, USA

First published 2005

A catalogue record of this book is available from the British Library

ISBN-13 978 0335 21388 7 (pb) 978 0335 21389 4 (pb)
ISBN-10 0 335 21388 X (pb) 0 335 21389 8 (hb)

Library of Congress Cataloguing-in-Publicaton Data
CIP data applied for

Typeset by YHT Ltd, London
Printed in th UK by Bell and Bain Ltd, Glasgow

For Fiona, Tristan and Daniel

Contents

Acknowledgements

Many people have contributed in different ways to the writing of this book: students, colleagues and family. Its style owes much to the contribution of students, from whom I have learned a great deal about making concepts and theories relevant. Many people alongside whom I have worked in the health service have had an influence, as have my current academic colleagues. In addition to those within my own discipline, who help sustain a stimulating intellectual environment, I have greatly benefited from the opportunity to work with others involved in delivering health programmes. I am particularly indebted to Julie Parsons, Karen Gresty, Andy Evenden, Graham Russell and Jenny Kevern.

I am grateful for the influence of my parents in helping to shape my thinking and values in many of the areas covered in this book, particularly on the impact of social inequality.

Finally, the biggest burden of ensuring the book got written has fallen on my own family: Fiona, Tristan and Daniel. It is they who are owed the greatest thanks.

Preface

As this book was being written, barely a week passed without media and political attention being focused on some aspect of health care. Very often at the centre of attention were the institutional arrangements of the NHS. Did patients get listened to sufficiently? Do they have enough choice? Who should make decisions about the availability of services?

Throughout all of this, a constant message from politicians has been the need to 'modernize' the NHS. Modernization can mean many things, but a key issue in these debates has become the opportunities available to patients to make choices about their own care and treatment.

Putting material for the book together, it became increasingly apparent that an important focus had to be the implications of this for professionals, at the interface between policy changes and individual patients. This is not a book about NHS policy, but it refers to many current developments to explore from a sociological perspective.

A literal meaning of the word sociology, from its Greek roots, is the study of companionship. More typically it is used to describe the study of society, social institutions and social groups. This is a broad canvas, and inevitably it has stimulated a variety of different approaches and methods. An early example, in the nineteenth century, was associated with August Comte, who believed sociology could emulate the natural sciences, establishing laws of society analogous to those of physics and chemistry. Few now harbour this ambition, but there remains a significant tradition that emphasizes the importance of scientific method and investigation.

Others argue that human society must be understood in quite different ways. This book avoids entering these methodological debates, but one of its objectives is to stimulate creative but reasoned thinking about the social relationships involved in health care. Good research evidence can help us do this, but so can other material. This is why, alongside examples from sociological research, the book includes material from other disciplines, including history, moral philosophy and social policy. The view is taken that the boundaries of academic disciplines should assist analysis, not impose irrelevant limitations. Rather than attempting to cover briefly a wide range of data and other evidence, my preference has been to be selective and to provide more detail and comment on a smaller number of sources. Frequently, this includes some quite extensive extracts from the original research studies or associated papers. Inevitably, it means many studies and examples that might have been included are not.

Comments are also included from politicians, journalists and novelists. Not all contributions may be judged equally valid in terms of describing how things actually are, but they can help improve our understanding of what changes are underway, and how these are viewed from different standpoints.

There are those who may prefer the philosophy of Mr Gradgrind, in Dickens' novel, *Hard Times*:

> Now, what I want is, Facts. Teach these boys and girls nothing but Facts. Facts alone are wanted in life. Plant nothing else, and root out everything else. You can only form the minds of reasoning animals upon Facts: nothing else will ever be of any service to them. This is the principle on which I bring up my own children, and this is the principle on which I bring up these children. Stick to Facts, sir!
>
> (Dickens 1989: 1)

In many health care settings there can be a range of facts to take into account, requiring judgement and expertise to achieve a balanced assessment. There may be a clinically effective intervention available for a condition, but if an individual patient does not wish to receive this, which fact is to count?

Even more fundamental are questions about the causes and origins of illness. In November 2004 Lord Lloyd, a former appeal court judge, announced the results of an inquiry into illnesses experienced by service personnel who served in the 1991 Gulf war. Governments since that first Gulf war had rejected claims that this revealed evidence of a 'Gulf War syndrome', but Lord Lloyd's conclusion, summarized in one newspaper report, was that 'veterans' feelings of being let down and rejected by the Government were justified. The damage to their health of having served in the first Gulf war was "indisputable".'

The report went on to note:

> The findings, though without official status, could prove politically difficult for the government which has consistently refused a public inquiry saying scientific research should come first. It has always rejected the notion of a syndrome, while recognising some veterans who were ill believed this ill health is unusual and related to their Gulf experience.
>
> (*Guardian* 18.11.04)

'Gulf war syndrome' is only one example of many long-term health problems for which origins are disputed. Explaining relationships between causes and effects is an important objective for many scientific investigations, but in the field of health and illness is made particularly complex by the large number of possible factors. It is no intention of this book to weigh the relative merits of different interpretations, but instead it starts from an assumption that many illnesses can have a variety of 'causes'. When we are tired or run down we may become more susceptible to infection, but would we describe the cause as the virus or bacteria we contacted or the state of our immune system? Both are implicated and, for the purpose of this book, it is relatively unimportant which might be assessed as the most significant. What matters more is how these different factors are judged and incorporated into everyday life and practices, by patients and professionals. In other words, it is with how people explain and deal with health and illness that this book is concerned.

One aspect of illness that features prominently is its relationship to the organization of society in which we live. The concept of 'psycho-social' influences on health is utilized to explore relationships between the social world and individual experiences. This is not to suggest that illnesses are mostly psychological in origin, but to recognize the significant contribution this can play. After all, it is not always helpful to make a clear demarcation between the state of our physical bodies and our social and emotional well-being.

This has important implications for how health care is delivered, a point referred to by the National Institute of Clinical Evidence in guidelines on the treatment of depression issued in December 2004. The report comments:

> The guideline draws on the best current available evidence for the treatment and management of depression. However, there are some significant limitations to the current evidence base, which have considerable implications for this guideline ... the most significant limitation is with the concept of depression itself. The view of the Guideline Development Group is that it is too broad and heterogeneous a category, and has limited validity as a basis for effective treatment plans. A focus on symptoms alone is not sufficient because a wide range of biological, psychological and social factors have a significant impact on response to treatment and are not captured by the current diagnostic systems.
>
> (National Institute of Clinical Evidence 2004a: 8)

In several respects this statement illustrates some of the underlying themes of this book. Health professionals work with patients within an established clinical framework, but this provides an inevitably narrow focus. Changes in the traditional relationship between patients and professionals are being encouraged; having possible implications for how problems are approached and dealt with.

All skilled work requires the use of judgement, and no book can provide definitive recommendations: what this book seeks to do is apply insights from the discipline of sociology to current issues and controversies within health care. An important strand running throughout the book is the centrality of the professional to the relationship between a state-provided service and those who use it.

My own thinking on these issues comes from diverse sources, as I have been fortunate to observe the NHS from different perspectives. My first degree, in psychology, and higher degrees in Industrial and Business Studies developed my interest and understanding of health care and its organization. For several years I worked as a porter in the NHS, when I was also active in my trade union. During the past decade and more, most of my teaching has involved nurses, midwives and other health professionals. My research has explored working relationships between different staff groups, in addition to issues arising from industrial and professional objectives of trade unions.

As an elected member of a local authority, I was for several years Chair of a Social Services committee, and for the past few years I have been a Non-Executive Director of a large Primary Care Trust. That role gives me insights into a spectrum of NHS issues from individual complaints to long-term strategic developments.

Finally, and most importantly, I have been a relative of patients requiring significant support from the NHS.

All of these experiences influence my thinking and outlook. These are reflected in the book, much of which differs from a conventional textbook. This is more a guidebook than a textbook. For instance, it does not include separate chapters on issues such as class, gender or ethnicity. These social categories are considered but within a structure that is organized around aspects of relationships in health care and the social distribution of illness.

Like any guide book, it is no substitute for the real journey, but can point to important features on the way. Its approach is one that seeks to prompt imaginative thinking about the social relationships in health care, rather than impart an all-embracing review of the discipline of sociology, or even its application to health and illness. For these reasons, I have tried to develop an argument running through the book, taking account of different perspectives along the way. The approach adopted may well not be shared by all, and other interpretations are available. Concepts, ideas and evidence about health and health care are offered as a framework within which current issues can be considered. Above all, the hope is to stimulate critical and aware thinking that might avoid a decline into simplistic rhetoric that currently dominates so much of public debate.

Part 1

Health care and the social distribution of knowledge

1
Health care and the 'sociological imagination'

A key focus throughout much of this book is the British National Health Service (NHS). Not the details of organizational structures, or some of the wider policy debates, but the means by which millions of people access health care and have contact with health professionals. Other contexts will be considered but the scale of NHS activity is unique.

- Every day nearly one million people will visit their GP.
- In an average week, half a million courses of dental treatment are provided by the NHS.
- In the course of a month, a million people will receive treatment as a hospital inpatient.
- Over a year, around forty-five million outpatient appointments will take place.

Beyond the NHS, seven million people are covered by private health insurance schemes. Independent sector nursing homes provide care and accommodation for over 70,000 people and, to take just one example from the use of complementary therapies, 3,000 osteopaths provide around seven million consultations a year.

Many individuals receive health services because of illness, but this is not the only cause. From disability to emotional problems, from vaccinations to pregnancy, there are many reasons why people find themselves dealing with health professionals. The term 'health care', in the title of this book, is intended to cover this wide range of activity – certainly not just what takes place in acute hospitals.

The aim of this book is to provide suggestions and examples of how sociological concepts and insights can be used to help think about important contemporary issues in health care. For that reason, it has a practical as well as an academic purpose, aiming to contribute to improving the quality of interaction between patients and practitioners.

Any attempt at applying the insights of an academic discipline to a sphere of practical activity risks failure on at least two grounds. The result may be judged to possess insufficient depth and rigour from the perspective of the discipline; and from a practitioner's viewpoint, it may lack adequate relevance and application.

It is tempting to avoid the risks entirely, particularly as many books currently available provide perfectly good introductions to the subject of sociology. More-over, many take as their particular focus the context of health, illness and health care.

What makes this book different?

The overriding objective of this book is to use sociological insights and concepts to stimulate thinking about health care: how it is delivered and some of the current challenges it faces. It does not attempt to provide a comprehensive introduction to the discipline, or to include all aspects of health and health care. Of course, this leaves it open to a third potential charge: that its content is partial and selective.

This is unavoidably true but selection of material for inclusion is neither random nor arbitrary. Instead, it has been determined from a view that health services and, more accurately, those working within them, will confront two fundamentally important questions in coming years. The questions are these:

1. What kind of relationship is needed between patients and practitioners, and how are inequalities between them to be addressed?
2. How do we respond to rising levels of illness, particularly those associated with chronic disease (recognizing its unequal distribution in society)?

Of course there are many other crucial questions facing the future of health care: from the implications of developments in genetics to issues such as the boundaries with social care; quite apart from matters of resources and funding. These are all immensely important but there is a rationale for selecting the two questions identified here.

A focus on inequality

Whatever organizational changes occur in the health care system, the experiences of most individuals using the services are shaped by the character and quality of their immediate relationships with practitioners. This provides the setting in which other issues arise and are dealt with. In the past, these relationships have frequently been perceived as unequal, with concerns about the 'paternalism' of health professionals coming to the fore in recent inquiries into paediatric cardiac surgery at Bristol Royal Infirmary and into the removal and storage of human organs at the Alder Hey hospital in Liverpool.

The Alder Hey inquiry report refers to the definition of paternalism provided in the *Concise Oxford Dictionary* as 'the policy of restricting the freedom and responsibilities of one's dependants in their supposed best interest'. Concerns about the possible consequences of professional paternalism were forcibly expressed to the Bristol inquiry by a group representing parents:

> Medical practice is essentially an intellectual pursuit. Being ill is a highly emotional experience ... patients are deemed incapable of deciding what is in

their medical interests. They become clinical material to which things are done.

(Redfern 2001: 23 281.3)

The encounter between a patient and a practitioner is more than a one-to-one interaction. It occurs in a setting that has already to some extent been structured: by expectations about roles and responsibilities; by differing access to resources such as technical knowledge; and by contrasting levels of authority. The importance of this social relationship, and the fact that current arrangements have been under challenge, requires serious attention be given to it and the type of change that may affect it. Although it cannot be the role of an academic discipline such as sociology to be prescriptive on alternatives, it can offer ideas and ways of thinking about problems to help clarify such thinking.

Much the same applies to the second question. Several current policy issues, such as those relating to the health care/social care boundary, and some funding controversies, are related to rising levels of chronic illness. The term describes that which is long-term and enduring, rather than episodic periods of acute illness. Its rising importance for shaping people's experiences of illness provides sufficient reason for regarding this as an issue of underlying significance. Furthermore, although socio-economic inequalities in health exist in most categories of illness, in few are they as extreme as in chronic disease. Considering responses to chronic disease necessarily entails addressing inequalities in health.

These two themes, challenges to the traditional patient–practitioner relationship and the uneven increases in levels of chronic illness, provide the basic structure to the book. A fulcrum on which this is set is the concept of inequality. One aspect of this relates to how technical knowledge is socially distributed, and the implications of this for power and decision making. Another concerns the social distribution of health and illness, and some of the consequences of this for health services. These are important questions for health professionals and society in general, and they are ones to which academic disciplines have a responsibility to contribute.

Themes of the book

To explain the approach being taken in this book, the following sections introduce themes that run throughout the book, presented in terms of what might appear as contrasting dimensions: theory and practice; the personal and the social; and facts and values.

Most bodies regulating the education of health professionals stress the importance of integrating theoretical and practice-based contributions, but academic disciplines such as sociology can be perceived as too theoretical and abstract. Connections with practice may seem too remote. A few comments are therefore required on why reliance on 'practical knowledge' may be insufficient.

A second point to consider is the relationship between the spheres of the personal and the social. The majority of health care practitioners expect to be working on a one-to-one basis with patients or clients. Sociology, in contrast, can be seen as concerned with more 'macro' issues of social systems and structures. Although this is not necessarily an accurate perception, there is a need to consider how we can understand interconnections between personal experiences and their social circumstances.

A third dimension is the relationship between facts and values. The distinction may not always be clear cut, as what counts as a 'fact' can itself sometimes be disputed. Nevertheless, sociology inevitably enters areas of debate where strong views can be held. These may originate in religious belief, political principles, or some other source, and it is no role of social science to supplant debates that ultimately revolve around the values people hold. Nor, however, should it retreat from these issues, simply for that reason. Instead, clarity is needed about the basis on which viewpoints are founded. Where this is lacking, confusion can arise about the grounds on which a proposition is justified.

Theory and practice

Julia Magnet, an American journalist living in London, with long experience of dealing with her own illness, found herself in a London teaching hospital. Experiencing what she regarded as inadequate nursing care, she later described what she believes is a crisis facing nursing:

> The real crisis is not about quantity – it is about quality. What was profoundly wrong in my hospital was that nursing – in its most basic sense, care – was almost entirely absent. To search for the solution in money, or recruitment, or bureaucratic restructuring is to miss the point. What we are dealing with is a change in the culture of nursing – the result of a modern obsession with status and self-assertion.
>
> 'I'm glad I trained when I did', said a newly retired nurse. 'I learned real things, how the body worked; now they learn airy-fairy things like how to work with other people. That should be part of your experience, not your training.'
>
> ...Nurses who went into the profession in order to nurse the sick feel dissatisfied (unless they are the lucky few who have escaped into more specialist niches such as paediatrics or intensive care). But after years of 'sociology and the NHS', the dissatisfied nurses can't articulate their dissatisfaction. They have been robbed of the language of compassion and had it replaced by union-speak, which picks up where university ideology leaves off, indoctrinating nurses in the dangers of 'racism in the NHS' or 'harassment'.
>
> (Magnet 2003)

Magnet's conclusions can be dismissed as superficial, and fairly wide off the mark, but her experience contains a message that should be heeded. This concerns the relationship, referred to by the recently-retired nurse, between training and experience. If these do not connect, there are dangers of seeing the contribution made by academic disciplines to professional education as irrelevant and a distraction.

Theories represent attempts to understand and explain the world around us. Despite that, theoretical ideas, and especially those generated in disciplines such as sociology, can be perceived as obscure and unintelligible. The response to the quip, 'What do you get if you cross a member of the mafia with a sociologist?' (an offer you can't understand) captures certain popular images of the impenetrability of sociological jargon.

In the second edition of *Fowler's Modern English Usage*, its author, Sir Ernest Gowers, admonishes those who adopt a writing style he describes as 'sociologese'. He applied the term to any writing 'which is over-complicated or jargonistic or abstruse', but a particular target was the academic discipline of sociology:

> Sociology is a new science concerning itself not with esoteric matters outside the comprehension of the layman, as the older sciences do, but with the ordinary affairs of ordinary people. This seems to engender in those who write about it a feeling that the lack of any abstruseness in their subject demands a compensatory abtruseness in their language.
>
> (Quoted in Burchfield 1996: 723)

A great deal of sociological writing does not fit this description, as Gowers acknowledges, but some does. Concepts not required in everyday language will sometimes be needed, and these may at first appear unfamiliar and complex. But their purpose is to help us organize our own thinking with greater clarity and rigour, not to confuse and disorientate. The issue of communication, highlighted earlier by Julia Magnet, can be used to illustrate this.

An example: communication between professional and patient

Consider the following two extracts, both taken from studies conducted in the period recalled with fondness by the nurse whose comments are reported by Julia Magnet. The first is an interaction between a nurse and patient on a hospital ward, and the second between a doctor and a pregnant woman.

> Nurse: There we are dear, OK? (gives a tablet)
>
> Patient: Thank you. Do you know, I can't feel anything with my fingers nowadays at all.
>
> Nurse: Can't you?
>
> Patient: No, I go to pick up a knife and take my hand away and it's not there anymore.
>
> Nurse: Oh, broke my pen (moves away).
>
> (Clark 1981)

> Doctor: How many weeks are you now?
>
> Patient: Twenty-six-and-a-half.
>
> Doctor: (Looks at case notes) Twenty weeks now.
>
> Patient: No. Twenty-six-and-a-half.

Doctor: You can't be.

Patient: Yes, I am; look at the ultrasound report.

Doctor: When was it done?

Patient: Today.

Doctor: It was done today?

Patient: Yes.

Doctor: (Reads report) Oh yes, twenty-six-and-a-half weeks, that's right.

(Graham and Oakley 1986: 60–1)

Much more recent evidence continues to suggest that failing to effectively communicate about illness and treatment are the most frequent source of patient dissatisfaction (Coulter 2002). As the Royal College of Surgeons admitted in a submission to the inquiry into paediatric cardiac surgery in Bristol:

> Proper communication between a patient and the surgeon responsible for their care is essential so that the patient can develop trust and is sufficiently informed to be a true partner in the decision making process. Unfortunately, this is the area of greatest compromise in the practice of most surgeons in the NHS and the source of most complaints by patients.
>
> (Kennedy 2001: 23 9: 283)

It can be easy to regard this as a consequence of failure on the part of individual professionals. Equipping them with better interpersonal skills may be seen as the solution. But look again at the extract from the consultation with the obstetrician. Why are the case notes and in this example, the ultrasound report, regarded as more valid than the woman's own account? (Even when she was describing results from the latter!) Why does the doctor put greater trust in the written report than in what the patient is saying?

These are questions that go beyond interpersonal skills of listening and into the area of the status that is accorded to different kinds of knowledge. This forms the focus for the next chapter, which explores this theme using concrete examples relating to health and illness. Having anchored this in a practical context, these issues are developed further and in a more theorized way in the subsequent chapter.

In common parlance, the words academic and theoretical can possess quite negative meanings. A standard guide, Fowler's *Modern English Usage*, refers to the emergence towards the end of the nineteenth century of one meaning of the word academic as, 'unpractical, merely theoretical, having no practical application' (Burchfield 1996: 12). During the course of this book, several key sociological theories and concepts will be introduced but there will be a continuing attempt to relate these to practical examples and illustrations. Claiming practical relevance is not the same as being prescriptive, and those wanting unambiguous, black and white conclusions will be disappointed. But this is likely to be the case whether you read the book or not.

The personal and the social

It is one thing to acknowledge the interdependence of theory and practice, but this alone does not justify the inclusion of sociological theory in the education of health professionals. Most professionals will spend their time with individual patients, so what value is a discipline that deals with much wider social and societal relationships?

This is where the notion of the 'sociological imagination' is relevant. Writing in the 1950s, the late C. Wright Mills, an American sociologist, reflected on the impact rapid social change had on people, causing feelings of disorientation and discomfort. Events in the private lives of individuals were very often the result of 'impersonal changes' across 'continent-wide societies', but as the distance between the personal experience and its originating factors grew, the connections became increasingly difficult to observe. Achieving a better understanding of how these were linked was, for Mills, the purpose of a 'sociological imagination':

> The sociological imagination enables its possessor to understand the larger historical scene in terms of its meaning for the inner life and the external career of a variety of individuals. It enables him to take into account how individuals, in the welter of their daily experience, often become falsely conscious of their social positions. Within that welter, the framework of modern society is sought, and within that framework the psychologies of a variety of men and women are formulated. By such means the personal uneasiness of individuals is focused upon explicit troubles and the indifference of publics is transformed into involvement with public issues.
>
> (Mills 2000: 5)
>
> ... The sociological imagination enables us to grasp history and biography and the relations between the two within society.
>
> (p. 6)
>
> ... Perhaps the most fruitful distinction with which the sociological imagination works is between the 'personal troubles of milieu' and the 'public issues of social structure'. This distinction is an essential tool of the sociological imagination and a feature of all classic work in social science.
>
> (p. 7)

In seeking to encourage a better understanding of the relationship between 'personal troubles' and 'public issues', Mills' view was that:

> Social science deals with problems of biography, of history, and of their intersections within social structures ... The problems of our time – which now include the problem of man's very nature – cannot be stated adequately without consistent practice of the view that history is the shank of social study, and recognition of the need to develop further a psychology of man that is sociologically grounded and historically relevant. Without use of history and without an historical sense of psychological matters, the social scientist cannot

adequately state the kinds of problems that ought now to be the orienting points of his studies.

(Mills 2000: 143)

The orienting points for this book, the character of the patient–practitioner relationship and the uneven rise in chronic disease, can both be better understood by applying a sociological imagination. On the first, professionals have various roles in assessing, treating and caring for a range of conditions, and these roles change and evolve. Partly this may result from the introduction of new therapies and interventions but other organizational factors can be involved. The roles of professionals are also subject to prevailing social attitudes or norms. These help shape the degree of authority the professional may legitimately exercise, as well as expectations about the way patients behave.

An example: the status of the patient
That the authority of the professional and the behaviour of the patient are not absolute and immutable is illustrated in a century-old account of the behaviour of a doctor in a teaching hospital. At a time when hospital treatment for many poor people was available only if they submitted themselves for use as teaching material, one doctor described scenes he had witnessed:

In every hospital recognized by the Medical Council as a place of instruction for medical students, the treatment of the patients is entirely subordinated to the instruction of those students ... Quite recently, I heard a railway signalman make a request. It was four o'clock and he had been waiting since twelve ... the visiting surgeon had given a long demonstration on him and was then discussing an entirely different question ... When the surgeon stopped speaking and began to draw diagrams on the board – diagrams which had nothing to do with the case in question – the man mildly and politely asked if he might go as he was wanted 'on duty'. He was instantly told to 'shut his mouth'. For forty minutes did the man wait and then the surgeon said, 'Dear me, how late it is! We must get on' and to the signalman: 'All right don't stand there, you can go'.

(Ferris 1967: 200)

Every time a patient and a health professional meet, their interaction occurs within a context that has already been socially structured. Not in the sense of being totally determined, but bounded and framed nonetheless. None of the one million GP visits taking place each week, or the equal number of monthly hospital out-patient attendances occur in isolation. The personal experiences of patients in one-to-one interactions encounters with professionals must be understood within the social and institutional relationships surrounding them.

The wider context

Although most of the focus of this book is upon the context of organized health care, it is important to appreciate the impact of wider, external factors. In some respects, powerful social influences can be likened to phenomena such as the moon's gravitational pull on the earth, i.e. being more observable in their effects than in their operation. Problems of directly observing the process does not mean, however, that the effects are not real, whether this concerns tidal movements or aspects of health policy. A key difference is that one is beyond the capacity of humans to control.

This can be illustrated by referring to the role of increasingly powerful commercial interests, evident in health care and society more generally. As many traditional professional powers have come under attack, it appears to be commercial interests that are achieving dominance. An example is provided by experiences of medical scientists working on establishing a genetic test for cystic fibrosis at St Mary's Hospital in Manchester. In 1994 the hospital was contacted by a Toronto-based company that claimed to own the gene, demanding a fee every time the test was carried out.

As it turned out, the company did not own a British patent and so the hospital was under no obligation to pay such a fee. However, in 1997 the European Parliament considered a directive that would enable North American patents to become valid in Europe, prompting the consultant in medical genetics at St Mary's Hospital to warn:

> Licence fees and royalties will have to be paid on all patented genes. In the future genetic tests for heart disease and breast cancer may involve the testing of fifteen or more genes each ... This will make genetic testing much more expensive and inaccessible.
>
> (Cited in Monbiot 2001: 256)

Nine leading scientists wrote to the journal *Nature* making a similar point:

> Instead of helping biotechnology to make a responsible and useful contribution to medicine and agriculture, the present directive from Brussels succeeds only in threatening the very basis of scientific research – free access to material and freedom to pursue promising lines of enquiry.
>
> (Dalton *et al.* 1997)

The Directive was eventually approved, with some amendments, after a major campaign in its support. Although much of it was fronted by organizations representing the victims of genetic disorders, substantial support was provided by the pharmaceutical industry. A single company, Smithkline Beecham, spent 30 million ecus on the campaign (Monbiot 2001: 257).

Explanations, causes and effects

The purpose of theory is to help us develop better explanations of the world around us. Settings in which professionals and patients interact are subject to many influences. Reflecting on the character of these is important for developing a better appreciation of the possibilities and limitations of such encounters. It is also necessary to consider the role of the social environment as a cause of illness and disease. At a time when considerable attention is being devoted to genetic bases of illness, professionals and others need to be aware of what are often described as the 'social determinants'.

A potential objection is that although these factors may be acknowledged as important for understanding causes of disease, they lie beyond the capacity of health professionals to resolve. The role of the professional is to provide treatment and care for the person who needs it. However, as concerns about disease prevention come to the fore, this distinction may become more difficult to maintain. One example is coronary heart disease, a condition figuring prominently in current national health targets. In the mid-1950s, an account of the relationship between this illness and occupations noted:

> the frequency with which those who have to bear the stress of industry become ill and die with cardio-vascular diseases. G. W. Gray writes that 'the death toll of busy men of affairs who succumb to heart disease in their forties and fifties is startling.' ... this problem has become so serious that many of the larger concerns insist on yearly medical examinations of their senior executives in order that these conditions may be diagnosed as an early stage.
>
> (Brown 1954: 262)

The social distribution of heart disease has subsequently changed and half a century later a government review of recent evidence on health inequalities explained:

> The death rate from coronary heart disease is three times higher among unskilled manual men of working age than among professional men ... Emerging evidence suggests that a cause of coronary heart disease may be work-related stress, particularly where there is high demand and low control at work. CHD in civil servants has been found ... to be more prevalent in the lower socio-economic groups.
>
> (HM Treasury/Department of Health 2002: 6)

No mention is made, on this occasion, of employer initiated annual medical examinations! The 'change in heart disease from rich man's to poor man's disease' (Marmot 2004: 25) is a profoundly important social transformation, and without disregarding the role of genetic factors, these should not distract us from aspects of life more amenable to change.

This is why an important strand running through much of the book draws on an approach towards understanding health and illness that is currently frequently described as a psychosocial perspective. This does not deny the physical nature of many illnesses but recognizes two important features. The first concerns the complex relationship between our physical bodies and psychological experiences. Dealing with this in any depth is beyond the scope of a book such as this, but much of its approach is founded on the premise that psychological and emotional factors can cause, or contribute to, the onset of physical illness. These psychological and emotional factors, experienced by individuals, arise in settings that also need to be understood in terms of their social dimensions.

Being ill also generates psychological and emotional consequences, in addition to any physical suffering that may be involved. Again, the precise meanings of these will be influenced by the social circumstances surrounding them.

Several discussions in the book, on issues such as the experience of illness and relationships between professionals and patients, draw upon ways of thinking about illness that emphasize these psychosocial characteristics. In much of the second part of the book, this is addressed in terms of the ways in which psychosocial factors can influence health and illness. Although a fairly contemporary term, it taps into a rich stream of sociological work, extending back to nineteenth-century writers such as Karl Marx and Emil Durkheim, both of whom are referred to in later chapters. As Brown and Harris observed in their introduction to a study into the social origins of depression:

> There is a long history of sociological concern with the aetiological role of psychosocial factors in medical conditions. C. Wright Mills in *The Sociological Imagination* argued that the relation of 'personal troubles' to 'public issues of social structure' was *the* central feature of all classic work in social science. Sociology has been concerned not only with the workings of social systems as a whole, but with the impact they have on individuals.
>
> (Brown and Harris 1979: 3–4)

Facts and values

An alternative to criticizing sociology for being 'gobbledegook' is the objection that it is merely 'common sense'. We can all have our views about the problems we face in society, so why on earth dress this up as a social 'science'? Again, an example provides a way of thinking about this.

In October 1987, the magazine *Woman's Own* attracted attention after carrying an interview with the then Prime Minister, Margaret Thatcher. The interest lay in the Prime Minister's claim that, 'there is no such thing as society'. This brought immediate rebuke from those who saw damage to society and social cohesion as a consequence of economic and political changes then underway. Critics pointed to rising unemployment, the virtual closure of whole industries, and the impact this was having upon many long-established and close-knit communities.

Others were prepared to defend the point Margaret Thatcher was making, arguing that taken in context, the remarks were simply stating the importance of individual responsibility. The relevant section of the interview went like this:

I think we've been through a period where too many people have been given to understand that if they have a problem, it's the government's job to cope with it. 'I have a problem, I'll get a grant.' 'I'm homeless, the government must house me.' They're casting their problem on society. And, you know, there is no such thing as society. There are individual men and women, and there are families. And no government can do anything except through people, and people must look to themselves first. It's our duty to look after ourselves and then, also, to look after our neighbour. People have got the entitlements too much in mind, without the obligations. There's no such thing as entitlement, unless someone has first met an obligation.

(Cited in Willetts 1992: 47–8)

The extract makes clear Margaret Thatcher's main concern was to emphasize the importance of individual responsibility. She is challenging the idea that society has responsibilities to meet individual needs, unless the individual has first done everything possible to address them. It is also claimed that a call for 'society' to respond is in reality a demand on government. In that sense, she seems to be saying, society is an amorphous and abstract concept. Only government has the means to act in ways that are being urged: and this is not the proper role of government.

If all that was involved were a few remarks made in an interview with *Women's Own* nearly two decades ago the issue might matter little. This is not the case, with the role of individual responsibility coming to the fore in many subsequent political and policy debates. This has especially been so in the area of health and social care. Willetts has argued that:

The real tragedy of twentieth-century Britain has been the way in which the state has taken over and then drained the lifeblood from the series of institutions which stood between the individual and the government. Gradually we have lost sight of the virtues of those institutions which thicken our social structure and give it a richness which is lost if it is just individuals facing a Fabian, centralized welfare state ... Big government undermines community and leaves us just as atomized individuals expecting the welfare state to do everything.

(Willetts 1997: 17–20)

If we regard society as representing the totality of social relationships that exist within a defined area, it is difficult to take seriously Margaret Thatcher's simplistic claim that it does not exist. However, a closer examination of what David Willetts is arguing in her defence suggests a rather different interpretation. The target appears to be not so much a notion of 'society', but rather the relationship between the individual and the state. Individual responsibility is being emphasized and the role of the state questioned.

Without disregarding some significant differences between Britain's two major political parties, on this issue at least there is some agreement. Writing in *The Spectator* magazine, soon after being elected as Labour leader in 1995, Tony Blair also took up the theme of rights and duties, claiming: 'the clear dividing line in British politics . . . (is) the notion of duty . . . the rights we receive should reflect the duties we owe' (Blair 1995).

Similarly, Margaret Thatcher's underlying emphasis on the role of the individual has been echoed in 2004 by the New Labour Secretary of State for Health. Acknowledging a variety of social influences on health, he nevertheless concludes with a strong statement on the importance of personal responsibility:

> The prime responsibility for improving the health of the public does not rest with the NHS nor with the government, but with the public themselves . . . All of us have a responsibility for our health and there is a growing recognition that we contribute as much to our health and wellbeing as docs the government . . .
>
> I firmly believe that the government should take a lead in addressing these issues. But I also believe that no government or doctor can make a person healthy on their own. Ultimately, that responsibility has to lie with the individual. Only they can make the choice to healthy lives, to change their lives for the benefit of themselves and their families.
>
> (Secretary of State for Health 3 February 2004)

An increasing emphasis upon individual duty, with a concomitant scepticism towards 'big government', characterizes much of contemporary politics. This issue matters for health professionals, for it is they who find themselves at the interface between the state and the individual. However, the manner in which the issue has been addressed by politicians tells us nothing about how these relationships are understood and constructed by people in their own lives. We learn, instead, about politicians' views about individual responsibility. This is an important matter of party political debate, but it is not an analysis of society.

Understanding society

In the course of this book, issues will be explored using a combination of theoretical concepts and empirical evidence. The latter is drawn from formal research studies, employing a range of different methods. Social research, for practical and ethical reasons, cannot adopt the laboratory-based methods used in some sciences. One consequence has been a proliferation of methods that seek ways of examining the social world, which provide adequate alternatives to the laboratory experiment. Some methods involve the collection of large data sets, through surveys and questionnaires, while others include interviews and observation. A distinction is often made between these in terms of quantitative and qualitative methods. However, it is not a matter of one being inherently superior to another: the choice of method should be guided by the question being pursued.

All research of this kind is designed to extend understanding and increase knowledge. In this sense, if not in the methods used, there are close parallels with the natural sciences. However, and this can apply to social and natural sciences, while the methods used may be rigorous and aim at objectivity, the research questions themselves tend to be prompted by a range of influences. These include the values we hold: what we believe to be important.

For sociology this can be particularly important for, as Mills observes, 'we cannot very well state any problem until we know *whose* problem it is' (Mills 2000: 76). What may be a problem for one person or group may not be felt in the same way by others. Likewise, the same problem can be seen in quite different ways.

Consider the following from a report in the *Daily Telegraph*: 'Long term claims by the 2.7 million people judged by doctors to be unfit for work now account for a majority of all pay-outs, which cost the taxpayer £16 billion a year' (*Daily Telegraph* 20.06.04). What is the problem here? Is it the fate of people deemed too ill to work; or is it the cost of £16 billion to the taxpayer? Possibly both, but we need to be clear about how this and other problems are defined. In a short study that examined different aspects of power, Steven Lukes points out that power is exercised not only when the view of one group dominates over another, but also when one group is able to determine how an issue or problem is defined in the first place (Lukes 1974).

Values and academic responsibility

Power relationships existing between people may possess no social or moral justification but simply reflect the capacity of one group to exercise authority over another. Discussing the consequences of an increasing trend towards subjecting human behaviour and decisions to rational calculation, Mills makes an observation that has continuing relevance for contemporary debates: 'Freedom is not merely the chance to do as one pleases; neither is it merely the opportunity to choose between set alternatives. Freedom is, first of all, the chance to formulate the available choices, to argue over them – and then have the opportunity to choose' (Mills 2000: 174).

To be able to choose which hospital to go to for a surgical procedure may be a welcome means of getting the surgery completed quickly. But this is not the same as having greater choice over which treatment should be available in the first place. The possibility of bringing more informed and negotiated choice into these matters highlights the fact that social groups possess different levels of power, authority and knowledge. Decisions made within these settings are inevitably shaped by this fact.

C. Wright Mills believed academics had a responsibility to challenge and question this status quo. He was sensitive to the risk that social science research problems can be defined in ways that meet the concerns of those possessing the authority and resources to commission research, rather than others who might have an equally legitimate perspective. No longer 'concerned with the battered human beings living at the bottom of society' (p. 95), social scientists who adopt this route find:

> Their positions change – from the academic to the bureaucratic; their publics change – from movements of reformers to circles of decision-makers; and their

problems change – from those of their own choice to those of their new clients. The scholars themselves tend to become less intellectually insurgent and more administratively practical. Generally accepting the *status quo*, they tend to formulate problems out of the troubles and issues that administrators believe they face.

(Mills 2000: 96)

The late Ian Craib makes some pertinent comments relating to this in remarks about the German sociologist, Max Weber. Aspects of Weber's work are discussed in more detail later, but we mention here that it stimulated Craib to note that the academic discipline of sociology 'involves the choices of some values over and against other values; it involves what are basically moral choices and the implication is that we need to elucidate the moral choice that we make. Very few sociologists embark on that enterprise' (Craib 1997: 52).

One cause of this reticence may be an anxiety that this would merely confirm prejudices that sociologists are weighty on opinion and light on fact. Emphasizing the results of rigorous empirical research can be an antidote to these conceptions but, for the reasons given by Mills and Craib, explicit statements of underpinning values are sometimes required. This is of particular importance in the context of health and health care, where moral views about the role of individual responsibility can be prominent. For this reason, conscious it may seem a little self-indulgent, some remarks about my own views and values are appropriate.

The value of equality

Politically, I am on the Left. That statement requires a little explanation, particularly as the left–right distinction is now held by some to be antiquated and irrelevant. I am unconvinced by that assertion. What I regard the term 'left' as meaning is probably best described by the Italian political thinker, Norberto Bobbio, who argues that the defining criterion for distinguishing left and right is the attitude to equality:

> When we say that the left has a greater tendency to reduce inequalities, we do not mean that it intends to eliminate all inequalities, or that the right wishes to preserve them all, but simply that the former is more egalitarian, and the latter more inegalitarian.
>
> (p. 65)
>
> ... We can then correctly define as egalitarians those who, while not ignoring the fact that people are both equal and unequal, believe that what they have in common has greater value in the formation of a good community. Conversely, those who are not egalitarian, while starting from the same premises, believe that their diversity has greater value in the formation of a good community.
>
> (Bobbio 1996: 66–7)

Bobbio develops a more sophisticated analysis, in a book that when first published in Italy topped the best-seller lists. Here it is sufficient to note the emphasis upon equality as a defining criterion.

That is a relatively easy part. It then becomes necessary to acknowledge that equality is unlikely to be achieved without some degree of planning and direction, requiring a significant role for government of some type. This has been a traditional goal for the Left, characterized in one form as representing a progression from basic civil rights (such as the right to a fair trial), through political rights (including the right to vote) to social rights (represented by the 'welfare state') (Marshall 1950). However, in recent years, the Right has argued 'that the implementation of social rights in the modern welfare state has undermined the sense of community by removing an individual's personal responsibility for his family and community' (Cameron 1996: xv).

This, as we have seen, is the view advanced by David Willetts, a Conservative shadow minister at the time of writing. I am sceptical about those who see solutions to social problems lying in individuals assuming greater personal responsibility. This is not because I believe people have no obligation to accept responsibility for their actions, but that is a different matter. My fear is that outcomes will reflect existing locations within the social hierarchy. In other words, demanding that individuals do more to provide for themselves may reinforce existing inequalities, rather than reduce them.

Being sceptical about currently popular arguments that the welfare state encourages 'dependency' does not mean dismissing arguments about the dangers of 'paternalistic' services. However, we need to consider carefully the character of these before assuming that the solution is simply to shift choice from the provider to the patient. An important point to note is that many of today's health and social care professions emerged and developed in the context of the welfare state. As the historian, Harold Perkin, has observed:

> Between 1945 and the early 1970s professional society reached a plateau of attainment . . . This meant . . . a society which accepted in principle that ability and expertise were the only respectable justification for recruitment to positions of authority and responsibility and in which every citizen had the right to a minimum income in times of distress, to medical treatment during sickness, decent housing in a healthy environment, and an education appropriate to his or her abilities.

> (Perkin 1989: 405)

Perkin quotes from Britain's first official handbook a section that appeared in annual editions for many years:

> In Britain the State is now responsible for a range of services covering subsistence for the needy, education, housing, employment or maintenance, the care of the aged and the handicapped and the nutrition of mothers and children, besides sickness and industrial injuries benefits, widows' and retirement pensions, and children's allowances.

None of these services has been imposed by the State upon an unwilling public. All of them are the result of cooperative effort between successive governments and the people whom they governed.

(Cited in Perkin 1989: 406)

Those circumstances may no longer exist but wholesale onslaughts on the alliance between the state and the professions need to be questioned. Shifting responsibility to the individual may be appropriate in many instances, but can also result in blaming the victim for their plight: 'Although "bureaucratic paternalism" must bear its share of responsibility for disempowering individuals, the view that rights are contingent on personal behaviour can evolve into a far uglier form of authoritarianism' (Sheaff 1997: 144).

More than this, I worry when some politicians challenge professional authority on the grounds that, being elected, they can claim to represent the 'people's view'. On questions of this kind we sometimes have to make our values very clear, an issue identified in the 1970s by the American sociologist, Daniel Bell. In a chapter entitled, 'Who Will Rule? Politicians and Technocrats in the Post-Industrial Society', Bell points out that: 'Decisions are a matter of power, and the crucial questions in any society are: *Who* holds power? And *how* is power held?' (Bell 1974: 358).

He goes on to argue:

The relationship of technical and political decisions in the next few decades will become one of the most crucial problems of public policy . . .

In the end, the technocratic mind-view necessarily falls before politics . . . what is evident, everywhere, is a society-side uprising against bureaucracy and a desire for participation, a theme summed up in the statement that 'people ought to be able to affect the decisions that control their lives'. To a considerable extent, the participation revolution is one of the forms of reaction against the 'professionalisation' of society and the emergent technocratic decision-making of a post-industrial society.

Yet 'participation democracy' is not the panacea that its adherents make it out to be . . . If individuals are to affect the decisions that change their lives, then under those rules segregationalists in the South would have the right to exclude blacks from the schools. Similarly, is a neighbourhood group to be allowed to veto a city plan which takes into account the needs of a wider and more inclusive social unit?

(Bell 1974: 364–6)

Given my commitment to equality, I am forced to acknowledge that restrictions must sometimes be placed on personal and group 'empowerment'. In many quarters today this may not be a highly popular standpoint, but I see it as offering the best chance of achieving a decent and humane society. We need somehow to achieve a balance that recognizes and utilizes the skills of professionals, while simultaneously increasing the control of those using the service. This is an objective urged in the report of inquiry into paediatric cardiac surgery at Bristol:

> We emphasise that we are *not* concerned to empower patients *at the expense of* healthcare professionals. The aim should be to foster an environment in which both patients and professionals feel that they are playing a mutually supportive role in the patient's care.
>
> (Kennedy 2001: 282)

This may be easier to describe than to achieve. And it will need constant renegotiation, so I see little point in searching for a universal model. Successful negotiations will require new skills on the part of professionals, and this is where my motivation in writing this book lies. My objective, to offer a practical guide for stimulating a sociological imagination, requires a considerable willingness to engage in what Mills describes as 'intellectual insurgency'. It demands that we think, question, challenge and criticize. Despite the many qualities of the NHS and the principles on which it is based, this kind of approach has not been a notable feature of its culture.

An additional problem is the shallow and petty nature of much that passes for political debate these days. All of us, whether as health professionals, academics and educators, or simply as citizens, have responsibilities to contribute to an enhanced debate. We must establish analysis and interpretations on firm ground; which is why good evidence is so important, and why we must go beyond our own personal experiences and beliefs. But we must acknowledge how these shape our perceptions of existing problems, and our ideas about possible alternatives.

Structure of the book

A dominant concern in the first part of the book is to explore the professional–patient relationship in terms of inequalities in the social distribution of knowledge. Inequalities in knowledge, and the different forms that knowledge takes, can cause patients and professionals to approach decisions in very different ways. Chapter 2 begins to lay the basis for considering this, opening with some remarks on patient choice. Noting the relationship between choice, knowledge and power, the controversy surrounding the triple MMR vaccine is introduced as a practical example of what can happen when expert views are rejected.

Another example relates to controversies surrounding the appearance of Bovine Spongiform Encephalopathy (BSE) among cattle, and fears of risks to human health. The two examples are used to discuss issues around public trust in experts, and factors influencing individual choice, whether or not this is supported by expert opinion. This leads on to a short account of the development of medical expertise, rooted in scientific reasoning associated with developments often referred to as the Enlightenment.

At this point, work of the German sociologist, Max Weber, is introduced. Weber was interested in understanding processes in modern society he described as rationalization, involving the increasing dominance of rational calculation in decision making. But Weber also pointed to the roles of values, emotions and tradition in shaping human action; influences that may have particular relevance for understanding attitudes towards health and illness.

This theme is developed further in Chapter 3, to explore different aspects of the status of medicine in society and lay attitudes towards health and illness. Weber's four orientations – rational calculation, values, emotion and tradition – provide the structure for the discussion. Examples are used to examine the role each can play in shaping personal choices and decisions, and the scope for conflict between different orientations.

Building on this, the focus in Chapter 4 moves on to examine different approaches to understanding some of the consequences of clinical diagnosis. An important concept in this chapter is that of medicalization, associated with claims that medicine has become inappropriately involved in aspects of life beyond its competence to effectively deal with. This introduces questions about the nature of illness, how it is defined, and commercial and professional influences that may shape this.

Chapter 5 develops earlier themes to explore implications for understanding encounters between patients and professionals. Particular attention is given to considering the inquiry reports at Bristol and Alder Hey. Each gave prominence to the notion of paternalism in identifying what went wrong, and this provides a theme for much of the chapter. Challenges to paternalism are considered in terms of the informed patient, the idea of the 'expert patient' and the patient as customer.

The dominant focus in the book shifts at this point. Paralleling the earlier emphasis on inequalities in the social distribution of knowledge, the second part of the book addresses inequalities in the social distribution of health. Chapter 6 provides a context for this, beginning with a brief historical survey of the history of infectious diseases, used to introduce issues around the multiple causes of disease. Comparisons and contrasts are drawn between clinical medicine and public health approaches. More recent evidence is discussed in order to consider ways in which dangers to health from the physical environment may be being replaced by those arising from social arrangements and relationships. Examples drawn from different settings are used to prompt questions about the extent to which health professionals should seek involvement in wider social influences on health.

After a very short historical introduction, Chapter 7 moves on to consider the social distribution of health in more detail. The chapter assesses arguments about whether health inequalities justify attention; raising questions about the role of professionals in delivering policy objectives. A framework is then introduced that provides the main structure for considering health inequalities: in terms of material factors, behavioural/lifestyle factors and psychosocial factors. The first two of these are discussed in this chapter, with evidence on the respective contributions to health of income and poverty, on the one hand, and lifestyle and behaviour, on the other. Chapter 7 also provides an explanation of the way in which the concept of 'psychosocial' is approached in the two subsequent chapters.

The first of these, Chapter 8, examines psychosocial influences from a perspective of social relationships and health. The chapter is organized in three sections. The first section explores evidence on the role of intimate and personal relationships in supporting health, before examining ways in which these appear to be changing in contemporary society. Discussion then moves on to consider the relationship between wider social support and health, introducing long-established literature on the concept of community together with more recent debates about the role of 'social capital'. The third part of the chapter moves wider again, to the level of society, paying particular attention to the relationship between social norms, individual behaviour and health. The French sociologist, Emil Durkheim, believed major social upheavals and the disruption of social norms can have detrimental consequences for health, and this argument is considered using his own study of suicide as well as more recent evidence from the former Soviet Union.

Chapter 9 moves on to discuss another dimension of psychosocial influences, those arising from the social organization of the workplace. This chapter is in two sections. The first draws on historical accounts of long working hours, and more recent research into coronary heart disease, to introduce arguments that a lack of control in the workplace has damaging consequences for health. These claims are discussed and related to the work of Karl Marx, particularly his use of the concept of alienation. The second section of the chapter continues the theme of control in the workplace by considering health care contexts. Particular attention is given to looking at the influence of traditional hierarchical institutional arrangements, and assessing the extent to which these have been challenged. This provides an opportunity to consider how experiences of both patient and staff are influenced by these contexts.

The two main strands of the book, inequalities in the social distribution of knowledge and of those in health, are brought together in Chapter 10. Inequalities in access to health care are explored in a way that raises practical implications for professional practice. A considerable part of the chapter considers claims that people with the greatest health care needs do not receive an equivalent level of service. Some evidence can appear contradictory, and a route through this is established by relating the discussion to previous themes around knowledge, behaviour and illness. Varying rates of access between social groups can be understood as a practical reflection of different social, cultural and material circumstances. Implications of this are raised in later sections of the chapter, which consider examples of suggested responses.

An attempt is made throughout the book to maintain a clear structure and focus on key concepts, linking these in ways that progressively draw out some of the implications. By way of conclusion, some final remarks are made that relate these issues to wider concerns about the role and responsibilities of professionals in the context of calls for greater patient choice.

2
Whose knowledge matters?

Patients, knowledge and choice

One of the most frequently heard words in current debates about health care is 'choice'. An opinion poll conducted by MORI for the BBC Radio 4 Today programme found 74 per cent agreed with the statement, 'offering patients a wide choice of hospitals will help push up standards for everyone using the NHS'. In contrast, the proposition that 'offering patients a wide choice of hospitals in the NHS will mostly benefit the better-off and better educated patients' was one with which only 21 per cent agreed. Eighty per cent believed that, 'Britain's public services need to start treating users and the public as customers'.

Opinion polls provide only a limited source of evidence but public demand for greater choice in public services is undoubtedly perceived by politicians. Tony Blair, the current British Prime Minister, has claimed:

> We are extending choice. Choice is popular. We are living in a time of new and unprecedented aspirations, declining deference, diverse needs and greater personal autonomy. The demand for choice today encompasses every social class.
>
> (Blair 2003)

Frequently allied with this emphasis upon the desirability of greater choice in health care and other public services is another objective: that of transforming the relationship between service provider and service user. In recent years, the National Health Service has received considerable criticism for being 'paternalistic', with the professional assumed to know best and failing to give sufficient regard to the views of patients. Prompted by an inquiry into children's heart surgery in Bristol (described and discussed in more detail in Chapter 5) the Department of Health pinpointed giving more attention to the views of patients as an urgent priority:

> Transforming the NHS into a modern patient-focused service is not primarily about extra investment or far reaching structural reforms. It means changing the culture and the way the NHS works, so that listening to, and acting on, the

views of the people who use it becomes the norm and people are helped and encouraged to make their views known.

(Department of Health 2002: para 9.2)

A nationally provided course for health care support staff, such as porters, domestic staff and others, is now available on 'customer care'. In the programme, the word customer is used to incorporate other work colleagues, as well as patients. It may be that much of the work of these staff involves responding to requests from other staff, rather than patients directly, but this perhaps illustrates some of the difficulties of applying the concept of customer to health care.

Nevertheless, it is being increasingly used. The NHS has established a project intended to improve the 'customer experience', an initiative that has been explained by its senior NHS executive manager in the following way:

> We are making good progress on improving health outcomes and delivering targets. Now we need to do better on improving patients' experience and staff involvement. We want to see the patient as a customer. We took a Public-Private Partnership approach because the private sector has more experience of consumerism than the NHS.
>
> (*Guardian* 3.7.04)

An implication of developments such as this is that the interpersonal techniques developed in other settings can be, and should be, transferred to health care. The specific assertion is that private sector involvement in developing a new NHS consumerism is important because of its greater experience in dealing with customers. This may be true but it raises some quite fundamental questions about the nature of health care, and the extent to which it is analogous to other spheres of consumer activity.

Far from being an abstract point of comparison, the issue lies at the heart of many current initiatives intended to change the nature of relationships between professionals and patients. Some of these initiatives are considered in more detail in Chapter 5, but prior to this we need to consider the concrete settings in which patients and professionals interact.

Being a customer

Think about the last time when you were a customer. For me, it was going to a shop this morning to buy a newspaper. It wasn't even just any newspaper. I knew before I entered the shop which title it would be. The previous occasion I was a customer was in a supermarket, and again I knew pretty well what I wanted before entering. More significant purchases can require more advice but we may choose not to rely exclusively upon the person from whom we are buying. We may suspect that salespeople receive commission, or have some other incentive to increase sales. Without actually distrusting the person, we understand that their role can influence their enthusiasm for selling the product. As customers, we are continually required to fall back on the prior knowledge we possess.

Desire for greater choice can very frequently be made as an abstract statement. Tony Blair's comments, for instance, present 'choice' as an inherently 'good thing' but with little clarity about what this might mean in practice. If the notion is to be a meaningful one, we need to acknowledge that patients and professionals bring different forms of knowledge into any encounter, in very concrete and specific circumstances. These may relate to a particular condition, investigation or therapy. A consequence of this is that health professionals can find themselves in situations where patients seek choice that is not readily available, or at least not within the NHS. In these circumstances, there is a danger of a gap developing between the everyday world of health care and the political rhetoric.

For Paul Beland, a midwife in Peterborough, the consequence of this conflict was his dismissal. Beland, with eleven years' experience as a midwife, was with a client, Louise Cutteridge, who went into labour at her home. He assisted in delivering an 8lb 8oz baby boy. Three days later, Beland was suspended by the Peterborough and Stamford Hospitals NHS Trust, on the grounds that all midwives had been advised that home deliveries were to be discontinued until further notice. He was later dismissed:

> Beland says he knew all about the trust's home birth suspension when he agreed to go to Cutteridge's aid – but, crucially, he didn't think it was sustainable. He believes that a midwife's first obligation is to a patient, not an employer. 'The guidance given to midwives is contradictory,' he says. 'It says we have a duty to our employer, but also a professional duty to provide care for women and it acknowledges that we would not wish to leave a woman in labour at home unattended, placing her at risk.'
>
> 'I was being told I couldn't attend a birth at home as a trust employee, but I knew that as a midwife I couldn't leave a client to give birth without professional care. My interpretation of this was that my duties as a midwife were overriding. But that's not how the trust saw it.'
>
> (*Guardian* 08.09.04)

A study by the National Childbirth Trust in 2001 found one in five women were interested in knowing more about home births, but only about one in fifty actually has one. Rates vary considerably. Compared to a national average of 2.5 per cent, for example, the rate in South Devon is 11 per cent. Cathy Warwick, chair of the midwives committee of the Nursing and Midwives Council suggests many women find expectations for a home delivery are not always fulfilled. Describing letters she has received from women, she recounts:

They say they booked for a home birth and were told they could go for a home birth and then, with just two or four weeks to go, they were told that staff shortages meant there was little or no chance that it could go ahead, and that they would probably need to come into the unit to deliver. It's very, very, very unfair. I think it's worse than being told from the outset that there isn't a home-birth service at all. That would be a tragedy, but doing this is dishonesty.

(Quoted in *The Guardian*, 8.09.04)

Conflicts of this kind can arise in many settings. They emphasize the need to think seriously about the issue of choice, and its relationship with the possession of knowledge. If we seek a better understanding of relationships between patients and practitioners, and how these might be improved, a starting point is to consider the basis of the knowledge and understanding that each brings.

To illustrate this in a more practical manner, the following section considers aspects of the controversy surrounding the use of the triple Measles, Mumps and Rubella (MMR) vaccine. Indicating how difficult these issues may sometimes be, this example also points to the importance of knowledge and emotions in decisions about health, illness and health care.

Knowledge, choice and the MMR vaccine

In 1996–7, 92 per cent of British children received the MMR vaccine by the time of their second birthday. Two years later this proportion had fallen to 88 per cent, to 84 per cent by 2001–02 and a further reduction to 82 per cent by 2002–03. By 2003–04 the figure was down yet again, to just 80 per cent. The World Health Organization recommends a take-up level of 95 per cent to provide 'herd immunity' but in some areas of the country, such as South-East London, the rate is now as low as 62 per cent.

Despite overwhelming official endorsement of the vaccine, a substantial minority of parents have not been convinced. Why is this? Is there anything to be learned about patient choice from this episode?

The MMR vaccine was introduced in 1988. Nearly ten years later, in February 1998, the medical journal, *The Lancet*, published an article under the category of an 'early report', entitled, 'Ileal-lymphoid-nodular hyperplasia, non-specific colitis, and pervasive developmental disorder in children'. This reported a study of twelve children aged between three and ten, who had been referred to a paediatric gastroenterology unit. As well as histories of abdominal pain and diarrhoea, all of the children had behavioural problems, diagnosed as autism, which included the loss of acquired skills such as language. In each case, these had emerged following a period of normal development (Wakefield *et al.* 1998).

A focus of the article was on the possibility of a link between the hyperplasia in the intestine and behavioural disorder. It was recognized that as all twelve children had been referred to a gastroenterology unit, and all had been diagnosed with autism, it was almost inevitable that evidence of enteric (intestinal) disorders would be found together with behavioural disorders. The important question was whether or not some kind of causal relationship existed between the two disorders – or pathologies – experienced by the child: one affecting the body and the other the behaviour.

Or was the emergence of the two conditions nothing other than a tragic coincidence? It is not enough to show that events *correlate* (that is, show a mutual relationship of some kind) to conclude that there is a direct *causal* effect of one upon the other. A student who increases their effort may achieve higher grades and also become more tired, but it would be unwise to conclude that the tiredness caused the better results. A more plausible explanation is that these and the tiredness were the consequence of working harder.

When early evidence is emerging it can be difficult to establish with certainty whether or not a causal relationship exists between different events. However, parents of eight out of the twelve children whose condition was reported in *The Lancet* article believed there was a causal link between receiving the MMR vaccine and developing behavioural problems. The parents of the eight children had all first noticed the problems shortly after the child had received the vaccination, in one case within a single day, and all were within the space of two weeks. Five of these children had also shown an early adverse reaction to the vaccination, including rashes and fever, and in three cases, convulsions.

Speaking at a conference in Canada in 2000 Andrew Wakefield, the lead author of the study, expanded on this aspect of his evidence:

> I was told by my mentor to listen to my patient, or the patient's parents. The answers you are looking for they have ... Having been contacted by parents interested in my previous research, I began to hear a strange tale ... that children, who seemed to be perfectly normal developmentally, began to regress quickly after receiving the MMR vaccine shot. These parents were told by their physicians that there could be no possible link between their children's autism and their bowels. But the parents knew better.
>
> (*The Observer* 22.02.04)

The report in *The Lancet* noted the parental concerns, and refers to other studies reporting the onset of autism following MMR vaccination. This leads to a conclusion that although no relationship was proved: 'further investigations are needed to examine this syndrome and its possible relation to this vaccine' (p. 641).

Although this hardly represented a definitive statement, it was communicated in a less tentative manner in many media reports following a press conference given by Dr Wakefield. Long after the publication of *The Lancet* article, media reporting of the controversy remained, at best, inconsistent – as can be seen in the following examples of headlines and opening sentences from three newspaper stories in a single month in 2002:

> **New fear on MMR**
>
> Scientists have found new evidence linking the measles, mumps and rubella vaccine to autism.
>
> (*The Mirror* 09.08.02)

MMR study finds no link between autism and bowel disorders

Children with autism are no more likely to have had gut and bowel disorders than youngsters who are not autistic, new research shows today.

(*The Independent* 23.08.02)

Blood test reveals MMR jab IS linked to autism

A revolutionary DNA blood test has finally proved evidence of a direct link between autism and the controversial MMR vaccine.

(*The Express on Sunday* 25.08.02)

The response of expert opinion

The majority of expert opinion meanwhile had taken a very firm view that there was no evidence to support this hypothesis. (More details on the following examples can be found on the Department on Health website). In the month following publication of *The Lancet* report, in March 1998, 30 experts brought together by the UK's Medical Research Council concluded: 'There is no evidence to indicate any link between MMR vaccination and bowel disease or autism'.

Similarly, in June 1999, a review by a Working Party of the Committee on Safety of Medicines of more than one hundred children's records where parents believed autism or bowel disease was due to MMR found no such link. By January 2001 the World Health Organization (WHO) was stating: 'WHO strongly supports the use of MMR vaccine on the grounds of its convincing record of safety and efficacy'.

In Britain, in the same month, a joint statement was issued by the British Medical Association, Royal College of General Practitioners, Royal College of Nursing, Faculty of Public Health Medicine, United Kingdom Public Health Association, Royal College of Midwives, Community Practitioners and Health Visitors Association, Unison, Sense, Royal Pharmaceutical Society, Public Health Laboratory Service and Medicines Control Agency. The statement read:

> MMR is a very effective vaccine with an excellent safety record ... All of the major health organisations in the UK support the MMR programme ... MMR is scientifically proven to be the safest and most effective way to protect children from disease ... We strongly recommend that children are protected with MMR and not left at risk.

April 2001 saw a further review of the evidence relating MMR and autism, conducted under the auspices of the American Academy of Pediatrics (AAP). This concluded that: 'the available evidence does not support the hypothesis that MMR vaccine causes autism or associated disorders or inflammatory bowel disease' (American Academy of Pediatrics 2001).

The dominant view was summed up in a leading article in the *Archives of Disease in Childhood* in September 2001, which stated:

There is no good scientific evidence to support a link between MMR vaccine and autism or inflammatory bowel disease; indeed there is mounting evidence that shows no link ... While the final decision rests with the parents, the evidence of the safety and efficacy of MMR vaccine is so overwhelmingly conclusive that health professionals should have no hesitation in recommending its use.

(Elliman, Bedford and Miller 2001)

Despite such 'overwhelmingly conclusive' evidence, take-up of the vaccine was falling. A number of factors may be involved but of considerable importance is the relationship between expert knowledge and that which comes from direct experience. The parents who gave their accounts to Andrew Wakefield and his fellow researchers were desperately trying to understand the cause of their child's autism, for which no adequate scientific explanation existed. They knew the autism developed after having the vaccine and a link between the two seemed plausible at least. Many more parents might regard this as a reasonable conclusion and be reluctant to expose their child to what they perceive as an uncertain risk.

Experience and knowledge

Direct, personal experience is immensely important for shaping our perspective on events but it can be partial and misleading, opening the way for poor decisions and choices to be made. One reason for this is that in modern society there can be so many events preceding a particular outcome that an equally large number of possible causal processes are potentially available. The extract below illustrates this, drawn from an explanation given by an elderly patient of why an offer of vaccination for influenza was refused:

Patient: I'm nearly 87. I've had flu four times in my life. And I think I've developed a sort of immunity. And I don't want to spoil that immunity. And that is why I don't have an injection.

Interviewer: Right. So you think that because you've had flu four times, you probably won't have it again.

P: Well, it's a good record, isn't it and I'll be 87 in July. Plus, I've got two other reasons why. I know somebody that got GBS from it.

I: GBS?

P: Guillan Barre Sydrome. You're paralysed. He was paralysed from there down.

I: Really!

P: Yes, and I've got a friend, up Grange Road, here, who has flu every 21 days for nine years because of a flu jab. Yes. She has flu symptoms every 21 days. She's one, the doctors have told her, she's one in I don't know how many million. So that's another reason.

(Prior 2003: 50)

This patient justifies the choice by referring to experiences of friends. However questionable this evidence might be, it is preferred to that offered by medical science. If account is not taken of why people arrive at decisions, there can be a failure to engage with issues that concern them, including genuine anxieties and fears. For instance, a parent who had chosen not to have her child vaccinated appeared on the BBC television programme, Newsnight, in February 2002. Interviewed alongside her, the then Health Minister, Yvette Cooper MP, was asked, 'If N. decides not to give her children the vaccine it would be better for them to be given the individual injections wouldn't it?' The Minister responded:

> The clear medical advice we have been given is not only that MMR is the safest option for protecting children against these deadly diseases but also that if we introduce separate vaccinations that would reduce coverage and not increase it. What we would end up with is more children exposed to measles, exposed to mumps, exposed to rubella and more children becoming sick and in the end more children damaged and dying as a result. *That is the medical advice we have been given and we have to stick with that.*
>
> (BBC 2002, emphasis added)

Here the Minister appeals to the authority of expert opinion that has already shown itself unable to persuade a sizeable minority of parents. The scope for differences of view between lay and expert perspectives is considerable, and it is frequently health professionals who find themselves at the sharp end in dealing with these. If patient choice is to be meaningful, how are these conflicts to be handled? A starting point is to consider the role of scientific knowledge in health care and briefly review aspects of the dominance achieved by science in explaining health and illness. This provides an important basis for considering a feature that underpins much of the relationship between patients and professionals: the role of trust.

Science, reason and the Enlightenment

Before the advent of anatomical investigation and an array of physiological, cognitive and behavioural measurement techniques, what evidence was available to assist diagnosis and treatment? In most cases, the source was the patients themselves:

> Endeavour to get the history of the disease from the patient himself. Begin to interrogate your patient. How long has he been sick? When attacked and in what manner? What are the probable causes, former habits and dress; likewise the diet etc., for a week before especially in acute diseases ... In chronic diseases enquire their complaints far back and the habits of life ... Pay attention to the phraseology of your patients, for the same ideas are frequently conveyed in different words.
>
> (American physician Benjamin Rush, 1745–1813,
> quoted in Porter 1999: 257)

This was a period in which health care has been characterized as 'bedside medicine' (Jewson 1976). Payment of fees meant that patients were the patrons of doctors and, therefore, really were customers able to exercise choice. With generally close interpersonal relationships between doctors and patients, its precise character was open to the varying demands of the client. This gave way, suggests Jewson, to a second form of discourse between patients and doctors that he describes as 'hospital medicine'. Lasting from about 1800 to the 1840s, a period in which the hospital emerged as an important location for medical care, this period fundamentally altered the doctor–patient relationship. Associated with the investigation of physical disease and its origins, the growth of hospitals enabled a shift in control from patients to their doctors. Finally, a third discourse, 'laboratory medicine' shifted the focus towards laboratory science as the dominant form of knowledge.

These changes were themselves reflections of new ways of explaining phenomena that is often described as the 'Enlightenment'. This involved a dramatically increased focus upon science and reason, seen as the engines of human progress. As Roy Porter, in a comprehensive survey of the development of medicine, puts it: 'Reason, proclaimed Enlightenment propagandists, would create a better future; science and technology, as Francis Bacon had taught, would enhance man's control over nature, and social progress, prosperity and the conquest of disease would follow' (Porter 1997: 245).

Francis Bacon, to whom Porter refers, lived at an early stage of the Enlightenment (1561–1626) but one of his more frequently quoted aphorisms reflects the emerging emphasis upon understanding and explanation: 'knowledge itself is power'. A later Enlightenment thinker believed this could profoundly alter relationships between people, opening the way for greater individual autonomy and independence: 'Enlightenment is man's emergence from his self-imposed immaturity. Immaturity is the inability to use one's understanding without guidance from another'.

Writing these words in 1784, the German philosopher Immanuel Kant advocates an approach to life that is anti-paternalist to its core. It is not sufficient to accept a view simply because it is expressed by someone in authority. Succinctly, he captures the spirit of the 'age of Enlightenment' with the phrase, 'Sapere Aude!' (Dare to Know): ' "Have courage to use your own understanding!" – that is the motto of enlightenment.'

The spirit of the Enlightenment was founded on a belief that the application of science and reason laid the way for people to exercise control over a world that hitherto appeared to control them:

> For the Enlightenment thinkers, all aspects of man's life and works were subject to critical examination – the various sciences, religious revelation, metaphysics, aesthetics, etc. These thinkers felt and sensed the many mighty forces impelling them along, but they refused to abandon themselves to these forces ... Through reason and science, men could achieve even greater degrees of freedom, and therefore ever greater degrees of perfection.

Intellectual progress, an idea that permeated the thinking of that age, was to serve constantly to further man's general progress.

(Zeitlin 1968: 5)

Science and scientific advance were central and fundamental to the whole notion of the Enlightenment: 'Science's key contribution to enlightened thinking lay in its underwriting belief in intellectual advance and its staking a claim to be the gold standard of positive knowledge' (Porter 2000: 152–3).

Science, illness and patients

The advance of science brought with it numerous technical innovations capable of providing new sources of information about the human body and its functioning. 'The stethoscope,' observes Porter, 'began the opening up of the living body to science and the medical gaze' (Porter 1997: 347). From the stethoscope, first described in 1819, other developments included the spirometer (to measure the quantity of air breathed, in 1846), urinalysis (1841), the sphygmograph (for recording measures of the pulse, in 1845), the sphygmomanometer (to measure blood pressure, in 1896) and various improvements in techniques for taking body temperature throughout the century. No longer was the physician reliant upon the patient's own account.

Subsequent improvements in diagnostic tests further increased the potential for the patient's own account to appear less necessary or important. The term holistic has appeared in many nursing and other texts, reflecting a desire to recapture an approach that considers the patient as a person rather than merely a receptacle for illness and disease. Benefits resulting from medical advance do not have to be ignored to also acknowledge that the dominance of scientific models of health care risks neglecting other important sources of information about the human experience.

The reality of many health care contexts is that professionals must utilize more than one form of knowledge, a point argued by Davies (1995) in a discussion on the changing nature of professional work. She suggests: 'Formal knowledge is put alongside other knowledges, leaving a considerable place for adjustment and negotiation in the light of a carefully acquired and detailed knowledge of persons and situations.'

Davies illustrates this with an account of an incident in an Accident and Emergency department, included in a report, *The Value of Nursing*, produced by the Royal College of Nursing:

We had a drunk in one night who was shouting and howling in pain. He was a biker who had come off his bike when it had hit a wall. You know how sometimes you feel about drunks – he was making all this row while the quiet ones lie still and bleed to death – nevertheless there was something about the abrasions on his face that made me think he must have had a real bump on the head, so I held his head and neck still while the other staff got the clothes off him and splinted the broken legs. Even in X-Ray he was cursing and trying to sit up. We put on the lead aprons and held him down. He was known locally as a drug abuser and we wondered if he really only wanted some pethidine. I made sure he got some anyway. The relief was instantaneous, too quick, still I'm glad we got it for him. It quietened him down and it turned out that he had fractured his neck; one sudden false move would have paralysed him.

(Charge Nurse, A&E, cited in Davies 1995)

The expression 'professional judgement' reflects the fact that differing kinds of information may be used to reach a balanced viewpoint. It involves judgement and is not simply the application of a standard formula or protocol. Accounts offered by patients may possess no inherently greater merit than one proposed by a professional, but each contain important information. One view on this issue, from a medical perspective, is provided in an editorial in the *British Medical Journal* that discusses alternative models of the doctor–patient relationship in terms of a contrast between paternalism and partnership:

Successful partnerships are non-hierarchical and the partners share decision making and responsibility. The key to successful doctor–patient partnerships is therefore to recognise that patients are experts too. The doctor is, or should be, well informed about diagnostic techniques, the cause of disease, prognosis, treatment options, and preventive strategies, but only the patient knows about his or her experience of illness, social circumstances, habits and behaviour, attitudes to risk, values and preferences. Both types of knowledge are needed to manage illness successfully, so both parties should be prepared to share information and take decisions jointly.

(*British Medical Journal* 1999)

The idea that scientific knowledge can replace all other forms appears less tenable today than was once the case, but this does not mean that every claim should be judged as equally valid. We need a better way of organizing our thinking about knowledge and the forms it takes, if we are to find an adequate means of describing differences between the knowledge of experts and of lay people. One framework for doing this comes from insights offered by an early commentator on these themes.

Max Weber and rationality

Max Weber was a German sociologist living from 1864 to 1920. Weber was interested in explaining what he termed 'social action': 'action is "social" in so far as its subjective meaning takes account of the behaviour of others and is thereby oriented in its course' (Weber, cited in Lee and Newby 1983: 174).

What he is stressing is the role of other people in influencing our behaviour. This, for Weber, distinguishes 'social action' from other kinds of human behaviour, whose origins may lie elsewhere. Weber wanted to understand the origins of social action: what drives it? Weber describes social action in four categories, although not suggesting these are entirely discrete and separate, for he saw that much social action has more than one influence. The important feature for Weber was what he described as the 'mode of orientation' that each category involved, a crucial aspect of which was the degree of 'rationality'. In his 'Theory of Social and Economic Organization', Weber describes the four forms of social action in terms of their 'rational' characteristics, a concept easier to illustrate by explaining the categories.

First, Weber refers to action that he describes as:

> rationally oriented to a system of discrete individual ends (*Zweckrational*) when the end, the means and the secondary results are all rationally taken into account and weighed. This involves rational consideration of alternative means to the end, of the relations of the end to other prospective results of employment of any given means, and finally of the relative importance of different possible ends.
>
> (In Thompson and Tunstall 1971: 140)

While there is no direct English equivalent to the German *Zweckrational*, it is sometimes translated as 'formal rationality'. In many respects it can be seen as signifying part of the Enlightenment ideal, with a superseding of religion and superstition as primary guides to action: 'It means there are no mysterious incalculable forces that come into play but rather that one can, in principle, master all things by calculation' (Weber 1948: 139).

Weber considered modern society had increasingly adopted rational goal-oriented action as the dominant form of social action, a process he described as 'rationalization'. In essence, the idea can be expressed in the notion of 'cost–benefit analysis', in which we seek to calculate the relative advantages and disadvantages of taking particular courses of action. It is rational in the sense of being calculative and instrumental, oriented towards achieving a specific objective. This stands in contrast to Weber's second kind of rationality, one where there is a:

> rational orientation to an absolute value (*Wertrational*) involving a conscious belief in the absolute value of some ethical, aesthetic, religious or other form of behaviour, entirely for its own sake and independently of any prospects of external success.

Weber had in mind here the kinds of action motivated by a sense of duty, honour, religion, personal loyalty, 'or the importance of some "cause" no matter in what it consists'. Again, direct translation from the German to English is not possible, but the term 'substantive rationality' is often used in its place. Here the emphasis is upon objectives as being ends in themselves, often being sought without calculation of the costs involved.

The point that Weber is making is not about whether or not the values or beliefs are themselves considered rational, but that action can be seen as rational when it is directed towards a desired goal. Craib gives the example that people may differ in whether or not they consider it rational to have a belief in God, but when someone does believe in God it is rational to engage in church-going, prayer and related activities.

Weber's standpoint is summed up by Craib in a form that is relevant for thinking about the social contexts of many ethical decisions in health care: 'We have to choose between ultimate values and there is no rational basis for that choice. Once the choice has been made, however, the actions that follow on from it can be understood as rational' (Craib 1997: 47).

As an illustration, most of us would want to receive a life-saving blood transfusion if circumstances required it. However, there are those, such as Jehovah's Witnesses, who regard this as unacceptable. The reasoning rests on a decision of apostles and elders meeting long ago in Jerusalem, endorsing a proposal from James that: 'We should not trouble those of the Gentiles who turn to God, but should write to them to abstain from the pollutions of idols and from unchastity and from what is strangled and from blood' (Acts, 15: 19–21).

Most of us are likely to feel no more compelled to adhere to this last injunction than to call upon a priest to pull down our house if there is thought to be disease within it (Leviticus, 14: 33–57). Our response will reflect the status we accord to different sources of knowledge but the example illustrates how values and beliefs can have powerful, possibly life-threatening, consequences.

Thirdly, Weber refers to 'affective orientation', especially emotional, determined by the specific affects and states of feeling of the actor: 'This might include automatic, uncontrolled reactions, prompted by emotion rather than tradition.'

In these cases, the action is carried out as an end in itself, not as a means, as when we might seek comfort from one another at times of stress or anxiety.

Finally, Weber considers social action that is 'traditionally oriented', the result of long-standing customs and tradition. Similar to emotional responses, this might result in virtually automatic responses to certain stimuli, and as Weber put it: 'The great bulk of everyday action to which people have become habitually accustomed approaches this type.'

For Weber, traditionally- and emotionally-oriented forms of social action lie 'close to the borderline of what can justifiably be called meaningfully oriented action'. By this he meant that they could be considered as almost automatic and, therefore, not primarily oriented by conscious or deliberate thought. For that reason he tended to give most attention to formal and substantive rationality; but in considering aspects of health, and how people respond to illness and incapacity, it seems relevant to consider all four of Weber's categories.

Although the historical period in which Weber wrote was very different to today, Weber's four categories of social action remain useful as a framework for thinking about how we approach decisions about health and illness.

Rationality and choice

The categories seem particularly relevant for helping us organize thinking around the idea of extending choice in health care. If this is primarily interpreted as involving the calculation of costs and benefits of different options (Weber's idea of formal rationality) then the implication would seem to be that we need help with our choices from those who can best provide the necessary information. This is likely to be of a technical, scientific kind, requiring the knowledge of a specialist expert. However, although the development of specialist areas of expertise brings many benefits, it also reduces the number of people deemed competent to make decisions. In a classic sociological study of knowledge, Berger and Luckmann make the point:

> I not only do not possess the knowledge supposedly required to cure me of a physical ailment, I may even lack the knowledge of which one of a bewildering variety of medical specialists claims jurisdiction over what ails me. In such cases, I require not only the advice of experts, but the prior advice of experts on experts. The social distribution of knowledge thus begins with the simple fact that I do not know everything known to my fellowmen, and vice versa, and culminates in exceedingly complex and esoteric systems of expertise.
> (Berger and Luckmann 1971: 60–1)

This is truer today than when it was written. However, highly specialist, technical expertise is not always what is needed. Sometimes, choices are based upon the values and beliefs that individuals hold, and in such cases this kind of advice may be of less help. Much the same is true if emotional concerns, or the influence of traditional ideas, are the principal factors shaping our thinking. None of this implies the role of the specialist is any less important but suggests that not all problems and questions are ones for which technical knowledge and expertise is appropriate or sufficient.

Nevertheless, there has been a tendency towards defining problems as technical ones and therefore subject to the kind of 'formal rationality' described by Weber. As C. Wright Mills pointed out, how problems come to be defined can be crucial for determining how they are addressed.

Writing in the 1970s, an American sociologist, Irving Zola, illustrated some of the social implications of defining decisions as ones for which technical expertise is required by considering the example of water fluoridation. Zola describes the development of political controversy around the issue of water fluoridation in the USA, with the question being put to a referendum in many states. This frequently led to the proposal being defeated. The response in several US states was to amend the state law to define water fluoridation as a public health decision, rather than a democratic decision. This enabled it to be handled by expert medical officers raising, argues Zola, crucial questions about how such problems are defined: 'Thus the issue at base here is the question of what factors are actually of a solely technical, scientific and medical nature!' (Zola 1972, quoted in Cox and Mead 1975: 183).

There is substantial evidence that water fluoridation has positive benefits for dental health, but the example illustrates that the boundary of what is considered a technical judgement needs careful consideration. The wider population may be less informed about the technical arguments but they will be drinking the water. In such circumstances, the question of whose knowledge matters is a significant one. Increasingly, however, the trend towards defining problems as ones requiring technical and scientific expertise has raised another important issue, one that became apparent in the example of the MMR vaccine. This concerns the level of trust that experts command from the public.

Science, experts and problems of trust

Science is implicitly assumed to be neutral, beyond the influence and distortion of unsubstantiated beliefs or vested interests. Such a view is reflected in a statement by the British Medical Association in the 1980s, describing the difference between medicine and 'alternative therapies':

> The work and approach of the medical profession are based on scientific method, defining 'science' in the strictest sense of the word, namely the systematic observation of natural phenomena for the purpose of discovering laws governing these phenomena … As an integral part of the society in which we live, scientific methodology is generally held to be an acceptable basis on which to set reliable judgements, free from overriding social values and political bias.
>
> (British Medical Association 1986: 61)

However, as was seen with the MMR vaccine, even where a broad scientific consensus exists, this may not be universally accepted as sufficient. The role of personal experience has already been mentioned but another factor with which this can interact is the extent to which experts are judged capable of providing all the right answers. A study in which groups of people were asked about the trust they had in public institutions found: 'The focus group discussions suggest that deference to authority or experts – for example the acceptance of Government or scientific advice on public health issues – is declining. Many participants simply do not accept that experts know the "right" answer' (MORI 2003: 20).

Examples of comments made by focus group members along these lines include:

> If someone said to me 'you can trust my committee or whatever, we're experts', I'd think 'yes, I can trust you to do exactly what you want and try to bamboozle me.'

> He came back with three pages of statistical rubbish, and he said, 'the traffic has not increased since 1992', which I find incredibly hard to believe. I mean I've lived there for the whole of that time.

> I think it's too important to leave to so-called scientific experts. There are scientific opinions just as there are opinions of ordinary people and depending on your training or your upbringing you will have a bias.
>
> (MORI 2003: 21)

It is an oversimplification to assume that levels of trust in experts and institutions are uniform among the population but the report concluded that, 'by far the most significant influence, without exception, is personal experience, closely followed by the experience of friends, family and other people'. Again, this can be illustrated with a few examples:

> It was a keyhole surgery job and I was very impressed. I was only in for two days and was walking again by the end of the week. So my only experience was really very positive.

> A cousin of mine went to his GP, he just fobbed him off with different things. It turns out he's got a brain tumour.

> I think the NHS is alright, because on two occasions I went to the hospital and it was alright.

The report sums up what is suggested as two crucial aspects of the reaction of interviewees:

> This reaction again seems linked to the powerful impact of personal experience and knowledge; local knowledge that people acquire through their daily lives and their own observations is enough to offset official information or advice where they come into conflict. It also results from experience of past mistakes; participants are aware that 'experts' were wrong about issues such as BSE, and that statistics can be manipulated to suit a particular viewpoint.
>
> (MORI 2003: 20)

The example of Bovine Spongiform Encephalopathy (BSE) is particularly relevant because it points to an extremely important aspect: the extent to which science is regarded as independent and impartial. Here we may need to move away from a generic label of 'science', to recognize that levels of public trust in scientists can vary between different groups. In 2002 the Royal Society commissioned MORI to conduct a poll on public attitudes to science which showed, for example, that while 88 per cent trusted cancer scientists only 44 per cent trusted government scientists. Government scientists were very much to the fore in responding to BSE, as is likely to often be the case with issues of public health.

Science and trust: the case of BSE

The earliest recorded cases of BSE date back to late 1984 but when they first appeared there was considerable doubt about the condition, and whether it had any relationship with other animal and human diseases. Two particular areas of uncertainty were the relationship between BSE and spongiform encephalopathies found in other species, particularly scrapie in sheep, and whether or not there was any possibility of it being transmitted to humans. The following account describes some of the process by which these issues were dealt with by government agencies, drawing on the Phillips Inquiry into the outbreak of BSE for much of the material used (Phillips 2000).

By 1986 the government's Central Veterinary Laboratory (CVL) was receiving reports of cattle appearing to show symptoms similar to scrapie, a disease found among sheep. These reports, submitted by veterinary staff around the country, prompted the head of pathology at the CVL to issue a memo which advised 'keeping an open mind' on the nature of the disease 'until we have more information'. However, the memo went on to point out that:

> If the disease turned out to be bovine scrapie it would have severe repercussions for the export trade and possibly also for humans if for example it was discovered that humans with spongiform encephalopathies had close association with the cattle. It is for these reasons I have classified the document confidential.
>
> (Memo from head of pathology at CVL, 19 December 1986)

A desire to maintain secrecy around the emerging information was also evident a few months later, in a memo from the Assistant Chief Veterinary Officer, in May 1987: 'Because of the nature of the disorder, its political implications and possible effects on exports it is essential that VIS staff must not, at this stage, discuss it with or consult workers at Research Institutes or University departments' (Memo from Assistant Chief Veterinary Officer, May 1987).

Public concerns and official responses

As public concern about the disease grew, the government established the Southwood Inquiry, in 1988, to examine all available evidence. Reporting the following year, the tenor of its conclusion was that, 'the risk of transmission of BSE to humans appears remote', and that, 'it is . . . most unlikely that BSE will have any implications for human health'. However, it added an important qualification: 'If our assessments of these likelihoods are incorrect, the implications would be extremely serious.'

This qualification tended to disappear when the report's conclusions were transmitted through more publicly accessible routes. For instance, in May 1990 the Chairman of the Meat and Livestock Commission issued this statement:

> I would like to take this opportunity to repeat the most eminent and distinguished scientists in Britain and in the rest of Europe have concluded that there is no evidence of any threat to human health as a result of this animal health problem.
>
> This view has been endorsed by the Department of Health which in its advice to health authorities, has stated categorically that, 'beef can be eaten safely by everyone, both adults and children, including patients within the NHS'.
>
> (Meat and Livestock Commission press release, May 1990)

Despite these assurances, public anxiety did not diminish, reflected in decisions by several local education authorities to remove beef from school meals as a precautionary measure. As the *Guardian* newspaper reported: 'Local authorities around the country removed beef from school menus yesterday, ignoring assurances from the Government that the meat is free from "mad cow" disease' (the *Guardian*, 16 May 1990).

This produced a direct and unequivocal intervention by the then Secretary of State for Health, Kenneth Clark: 'The Health Secretary yesterday attacked the "idiotic decisions" to ban beef in schools and poured scorn on "crazy scare stories" which claimed that BSE could be dangerous to humans . . . "It is a pity that the people responsible for education have so little regard for medical science." ' (*Guardian*, 23 May 1990).

BSE provides an example of scientific understanding being shaped, not solely by the pursuit of knowledge but by the wider political and commercial context. This includes the economic interests of certain groups, often expressed as a national economic interest, rather than of a more sectional character. The inquiry into BSE illustrates how these interests and concerns influenced the way in which BSE was constructed as a problem.

Commercial interests and medicine

Similar claims about the role of commercial interests shaping scientific research have been made in the area of pharmaceuticals. Concerns that pharmaceutical companies abuse their position to achieve favourable scientific reports in medical journals have been expressed by Richard Horton, editor of *The Lancet*:

> Pharmaceutical companies have found a way to circumvent the protective norms of peer-review. In many cases, they are able to seed the research literature with weak science that they use to promote their products to physicians. Even what may seem like good research studies can hide sinister scenarios of bad news. Clinical trialists, for example, can begin with the goal of studying one outcome, but, when that result is less favourable than the sponsor would have liked, scientists may then choose (or be forced) to report a different, more positive, outcome.
>
> (*The Independent* 21.09.04)

David Healy, director of the Department of Psychological Medicine at the University of Bangor, has claimed there is now a crisis for 'evidence-based medicine':

> It is a crisis that stems from the fact that the marketing – as opposed to the sales – departments of some companies that accept that clinicians are primarily influenced by evidence, have, over the past 20 years, set about providing selective evidence in the best journals and with the best authors . . .
>
> This is an issue that goes beyond medicine and science. A great deal of the use of drugs such as the SSRIs in both children and adults appears to have more to do with what can be viewed as efforts to manage risks or enhance ourselves rather than with traditional efforts to treat disease. The promise of the new

biology lies in just these areas of risk management or enhancement as we seek to better understand who we are. The data that stem from biological and especially genetic sources will shed light on our attitudes and aptitudes and on many aspects of how we govern ourselves, from our proclivities to particular political or religious orientations through to our physical and mental abilities. But these data will for the most part be owned by pharmaceutical companies.

(Healy 2004: 20–1)

Whether the issue is one of identifying a potential health risk or the development of a new drug, alongside differing technical assessments of levels of risk and benefits, lie substantial economic and commercial interests. These provide powerful forces setting the contours upon which problems are presented and perceived. There seems to be increasing awareness of these influences, in some cases contributing to a wider scepticism about the impartiality of science. As trust in science diminishes, many people may prefer to rely on knowledge derived from their own experience, or that of others around them.

To explore this further, the next chapter examines some of the problems and limits that professional knowledge based on scientific principles confronts. Using the four 'orientations' suggested by Weber, the chapter considers the status of scientific knowledge in terms of conflicts between values and instrumental calculation; the role of emotions; and traditional and cultural influences.

3
Science, values, emotion and tradition

Despite attempts to subject an increasing range of problems and decisions to rational calculation, many do not lend themselves readily to this kind of process. This is especially so in the field of health care. For example:

- Is carrying out more surgical procedures a greater priority than developing mental health services?
- Are services for children more important than those for older people?
- How is the importance of speech and language therapy to be weighed against the need to develop oncology services?
- What relative importance should be given to services for those people with physical disabilities as opposed to those with learning disabilities?
- Should occupational therapy services have an equal claim to resources as maternity services?

The list could go on. A cost–benefit type calculation may be used to assess some options, taking account of numbers of patients involved, degree of incapacity, and suchlike. But ultimately these are not questions that can be determined wholly by formal calculation. It is what Weber had in mind when he referred to substantive rationality, founded upon beliefs, values or ideals rather than calculative, formal rationality. As Ian Craib has put it:

> Substantive rationality cannot be understood simply in terms of rational calculation – it concerns the things we value. A high level of formal rationality tends to enter into conflict, or at least tension with a high level of substantive rationality.
>
> (Craib 1997: 124)

Too great a focus on efficiency and effectiveness can distract us from considering what we really believe to be the most important goals. There can also be a tendency to reduce all questions to one of measurement and calculation, allowing costs and benefits to be identified more easily. Many government performance targets, such as those for reducing waiting lists, are intended to provide a quantifiable indicator of performance but cannot measure the relative importance of this goal against others.

This reflects an aspect of modern life pursued by several writers, a focus on what is sometimes termed 'instrumental rationality', where the value of things is subject to increasing analysis and measurement. Charles Taylor, a prominent moral philosopher, describes the problem of instrumental rationality as a 'massively important phenomenon of the modern age':

> No doubt sweeping away the old orders has immensely widened the scope of instrumental reason. Once society no longer has a sacred structure, once social arrangements and modes of action are no longer grounded in the order of things or the will of God, they are in a sense up for grabs. They can be redesigned with their consequences for the happiness and well-being of individuals as our goal. The yardstick that henceforth applies is that of instrumental reason. Similarly, once the creatures that surround us lose the significance that accrued to their place in the chain of being, they are open to being treated as raw materials or instruments for our projects.
>
> In one way this change has been liberating. But there is also a widespread unease that instrumental reason has not only enlarged its scope but also threatens to take over our lives. The fear is that things that ought to be determined by other criteria will be decided in terms of efficiency or 'cost benefit' analysis, that the independent aims that ought to be guiding our lives will be eclipsed by demands to maximise output.
>
> (Taylor 1991: 5)

Values and utilitarian calculation

As Taylor suggests, attempts are sometimes made to subject questions that simply are not resolvable through a cost–benefit analysis to this type of calculation. Charles Dickens had this approach in his sights in the novel *Hard Times*, intended as an assault on the philosophical position known as utilitarianism that gained considerable influence in the nineteenth century. To be utilitarian, as defined by the Oxford English Dictionary, is to 'regard the greatest good or happiness of the greatest number as the chief consideration or rule of morality'.

Decisions taken relating to health care may relate only indirectly to happiness but, as Butler points out, the guiding principle is much the same: 'the right and rational course of action in a situation where resources are insufficient to maximise the health of *individuals* is to maximize the health of the population or group *as a whole*' (Butler 1999: 135).

This has an obvious and potentially very important implication for health professionals. Decisions that produce the greatest benefit for the population as a whole may not be the best outcome for every individual or group within that population. With a few exceptions, such as public health specialists, professionals tend to deal with individuals, not populations. Utilitarian approaches have a different starting point and consequently may arrive at different conclusions about what course of action should be adopted.

Another way to describe approaches that judge actions in terms of their outcomes is as 'consequentialist'. Those taking a consequentialist position are likely to defend a particular course of action on the grounds of its anticipated *consequences*, rather than basing this on a moral view of the action itself. Some people, for instance, argue that the detrimental social and emotional consequences of forcing a mother to have an unwanted child justify termination of the pregnancy. Others take a view that, unless the mother's physical health is in serious jeopardy, or in exceptional circumstances such as rape, abortion is morally wrong as it involves taking the life of another. This type of position, in contrast to consequentialist arguments, is known as a deontological theory. The action is being judged for itself, not for its consequences.

Within the field of health care there are many examples where responses to interventions may be influenced by a sense of moral or other duty. For example: rejection of abortion by Roman Catholics; refusal of a blood transfusion by Jehovah Witnesses; and various requirements on rituals to follow at the time of death. In a range of settings, particularly in contexts concerning the beginning and end of life (from issues as varied as stem-cell research to euthanasia), views about the inherent rightness or wrongness of actions will vary. These differences can be debated and argued over, as they should be, but it can be difficult if not impossible to resolve them by rational calculation.

This is not always appreciated. As Sheila Hillier, in a discussion on rationalization and modern health care systems, observes: 'In Weber's view, the danger is that problems which are questions of value (wertrationalitat) become defined as technical questions (zweckrationalitat)' (Hiller 1987: 198). This, in part, was what the American sociologist Daniel Bell is referring to in his book, *The Coming of Post-Industrial Society*, when discussing the role of the 'technocrat', someone who possesses authority that is based on their technical competence (Bell 1974). Bell foresaw an increasing role for technocratic expertise but, as mentioned in the previous chapter, was aware that this might sometimes come into conflict with popular desires and sentiments.

Interestingly, many disputes between politicians about health care in Britain today have become ones of technocratic and managerial problems rather than underlying values. New Labour has made a virtue out of its concern for identifying 'what works', rather than attachment to ideological values and beliefs. But as Bell points out, there is much that lies beyond technical expertise. An impassioned plea to recognize the dangers of dealing with all questions as if they were technical ones, of treating every problem as if it can be solved by cost–benefit analysis, was made in 1990 by the then Chief Rabbi-elect, Jonathan Sacks. Taking as his theme, 'The Persistence of Faith', Sacks foresaw a society increasingly dominated by 'economic calculation, the endless solving of technical problems, environmental concerns, and the satisfaction of sophisticated consumer demands'. However, he warns, 'The human being as consumer neither is, nor can be, all we are, and a social system built on that premise will fail.'

He went on to argue:

Modernity is the transition from fate to choice. At the same time it dissolves the commitments and loyalties that once lay behind our choices. Technical reason has made us masters of matching means to ends. But it has left us inarticulate as to why we should choose one end rather than another ... Now we choose because we choose. Because it is what we want; or it works for us; or it feels right for me. Once we have dismantled a world in which larger virtues held sway, what is left are success and self-expression, the key values of an individualist culture.

But can a society survive on so slender a moral base? It is a question that was already raised in the nineteenth century by figures like Alexis de Tocqueville and Max Weber, who saw most clearly the connection between modern liberal democracies and Judaeo-Christian tradition ...

Max Weber delivered the famous prophetic warning that the cloak of material prosperity might eventually become like an iron cage. It was already becoming an end in itself, and other values were left, in his words, 'like the ghost of dead religious beliefs'. Once capitalism consumed its religious foundations, both men feared the consequences.

The stresses of a culture without shared meanings are already mounting, and we have yet to count the human costs. We see them in the move from a morality of self-imposed restraint to one in which we increasingly rely on law to protect us from ourselves. In the past, disadvantaged groups could find in religion what Karl Marx called 'the feelings of a heartless world'. A purely economic order offers no such consolations. A culture of success places little value on the unsuccessful.

The erosion of those bonds of loyalty and love which religion undergirded has left us increasingly alone in an impersonal economic and social system. Emile Durkheim was the first to give this condition a name. He called it anomie: the situation in which individuals have lost their moorings in a collective order.

(Quoted in Bocock and Thompson 1992: 327–8)

Many would challenge a claim that recognition of the importance of social bonds between people necessarily has a religious basis. Humanists, for example, could point to ethically-based principles that require no religious faith or belief. That aside, Sacks is identifying issues that have reverberated throughout modern history. These issues can be brought into a sharper and current focus by introducing a practical example, to demonstrate how a question can be approached in terms of 'cost–benefit analysis', or from the point of view of underlying values and beliefs.

An example of 'personal care'

This example returns to the issue introduced in Chapter 1, about individual responsibility for meeting welfare needs. Specifically, it concerns the type of needs that must exist before the state accepts responsibility for meeting them. The issue is one that has come to prominence, particularly in the context of a substantial decline in the NHS provision of long-term care. This decline has occurred over a long period and is still continuing, as indicated in the decreasing numbers of NHS beds available for specialties such as older people, and people with mental illness or learning disability (see Table 1.1).

Many of these groups of patients were defined as requiring 'social' rather than 'health' care. This led to a considerable growth in the provision of nursing and residential care but unlike the NHS, these services are not automatically received free at the point of use. Local social service authorities have responsibilities for assessing need and where this is judged to require residential care, financial support can be provided. However, this is subject to a means test and depending on the person's financial means, they may be required to make a contribution towards the cost of their care.

Table 1.1 Average daily number of available NHS beds by sector (thousands)

Sector	1995–6	1996–7	1997–8	1998–9	1999–2000	2000–1	2001–2
Geriatric	34	32	30	29	28	28	28
Mental illness	39	38	37	36	34	34	33
Learning disability	13	10	8	7	7	6	6

Source: Department of Health (2003)

There are historical reasons why these two frameworks, one relating to the NHS and the other to local government, developed as they did. But as NHS long-term care provision contracted, the consequences became more and more apparent. Complaints began to be raised that the system was anomalous, as an individual receiving free care in the NHS who then transferred to a nursing home would find themselves required to pay (subject to the means test) for services they had received without charge in the NHS.

With the issue becoming increasingly contentious during the 1990s, the Labour Party promised that, if elected, it would establish a Royal Commission to examine the problem and make recommendations. Following Labour's election success in 1997, this was done and the Royal Commission reported in 1999. A wide range of issues were covered in the report but on the matter of where the responsibilities of the individual and the state for funding care should be set, the Commission recommended a new approach.

This involved moving from an approach that emphasized the distinction between 'health' and 'social' care and introducing a new notion of 'personal care'. The Royal Commission was seeking to establish criteria in terms of the tasks performed, rather than the institutional setting in which they took place. This can best be explained by quoting the relevant section from the Royal Commission report:

6.43 By 'personal care' in this option the Commission mean the care needs which give rise to the major additional costs of frailty or disability associated with old age. We deliberately do not use the term 'health care' or 'social care' because of the confusion which now surrounds those terms and their association with particular agencies or forms of funding. Personal care is care that directly involves touching a person's body (and therefore incorporates issues of intimacy, personal dignity and confidentiality), and is distinct both from treatment/therapy (a procedure deliberately intended to cure or ameliorate a pathological condition) and from indirect care such as home-help or the provision of meals. This type of care is the main source of contention in the debate about the distinction between health care and social care. It falls within the internationally recognised definition of nursing, but may be delivered by many people who are not nurses, in particular by care assistants employed by social services departments or agencies.

6.44 Personal care, because it directly involves touching a person's body, incorporates issues of intimacy, personal dignity and confidentiality. Because of risks associated with poor personal care (e.g. risks of infection or skin breakdown), it is important that when the level or type of care needed becomes greater than can normally be provided at home by a relative or informal carer, careful assessment is made of how best it can be provided and by whom. It, therefore, differs qualitatively from living costs and housing costs. In recommending that personal care should be exempted from means testing, we are not recommending that this should happen on demand. Far from it, we have stressed throughout our report the importance of proper assessment of need.

Definition of Personal Care

Personal care would cover all direct care related to:

- personal toilet (washing, bathing, skin care, personal presentation, dressing and undressing and skin care);

- eating and drinking (as opposed to obtaining and preparing food and drink);

- managing urinary and bowel functions (including maintaining continence and managing incontinence);

- managing problems associated with immobility;

- management of prescribed treatment (e.g. administration and monitoring medication);

- behaviour management and ensuring personal safety (for example, for those with cognitive impairment – minimising stress and risk).

(Sutherland 1999)

The government rejected this recommendation. In its response to the Royal Commission report, it stated:

2.6 The main report of the Royal Commission recommended that 'personal care', which includes nursing care and some social care tasks such as help with bathing, should be funded from general taxation, subject to an assessment of need. At the moment, this is usually provided on a means-tested basis through local councils, so people who are least able to pay receive it free. As a result, three-quarters of those in residential or nursing care already get some or all of their personal care costs met from public funds. Making personal care free for everyone carries a very substantial cost, both now and in the future. It would consume most of the additional resources we plan to make available for older people through the NHS Plan. Yet it would not necessarily improve services as the Note of Dissent to the Royal Commission's report makes clear. It does not help the least well off. We have not followed this recommendation because we believe our alternative proposals to improve standards of care and fair access to services will generate more important benefits of health and independence for all older people, now and in the future.

2.7 Our investment in intermediate care services and in other preventive and rehabilitative services, such as community equipment, is fundamentally geared towards restoring older people's independence, particularly after an acute illness, or a fall, or some other crisis. This major investment will mean that more people will be able to continue living independent lives in their home communities rather than entering residential care. Where people need to enter residential care for a short time, our intended changes to the charging rules will help ease the pressure on people to sell their own homes against their wishes and will lessen the burden of care costs. This targeting of resources will provide a sustainable framework for future generations. It will ease the financial burdens on older people and their families, and drive up standards for everyone.

(The government's response to the Royal Commission
on Long Term Care, July 2000)

The government proposed that 'nursing care' rather than 'personal care' should be exempt from means testing. The subsequent Health and Social Care Act 2001 defines nursing care, in a care or nursing home, as the registered nurse contribution to providing, planning and supervising care in a nursing home setting. It does not include any time spent by other personnel, such as care assistants, who may be involved in providing care, although it would include any time spent by nurses in monitoring or supervising the care that is delegated to others. This embraces a much narrower range of care activity than that which would be included within the definition of personal care.

A different policy was adopted in Scotland, where the Parliament took the decision to implement the Royal Commission's recommendations. However, the argument persists as to whether this represents the best use of resources, with some suggesting that it has meant Scotland has been unable to develop home-based care to the same extent as in England.

The Royal Commission's argument, one that might be described as the deontological case, is based on the view that a person whose needs are so great that they cannot feed or bath themselves unaided, or go to the toilet without assistance, should receive state-funded services as a right. The counter-view, which can be described as the consequentialist case, points to the fact that spending resources in this way deprives other services of the necessary investment, having detrimental results on the care received by many more people living at home.

Estimates of future costs of long-term care for older people suggest that public expenditure would have to rise from £8.8 billion in 2000 to £35.46 billion in 2050. However, if free personal care were to be introduced, there would be an immediate rise to £10.3 billion, increasing to £42.6 billion by 2050 (Wittenberg *et al.* 2004).

Should a case be built on the fundamental values an individual believes to be right? Or is action to be taken only after calculating the best way of using finite resources? This includes taking account of what is sometimes termed the opportunity cost, that which you cannot do as a result of the chosen action. In England, the government decided to make a utilitarian calculation about how to secure the greatest benefit for the greatest number. An entirely rational decision, but one that may not accord with what many people judge to be right. The potential for conflict between utilitarian approaches and those that take absolute rights of individuals as a starting point can be significant. Sometimes this arises between policy experts and the public, with decisions justified on 'cost–benefit' terms being perceived as unfair and unjust. As the point of direct contact between the state and the patient, professionals can find themselves caught in the tension between the two approaches.

The National Health Service, as with many other health care systems internationally, has witnessed the increasing use of methods designed to improve service planning and performance management, and increase efficiency. These can often result in significant service changes, justified by the claim that they represent a better use of available resources. Sometimes there can be detrimental consequences for particular individuals or groups. In such circumstances, some employing organizations may expect staff to demonstrate loyalty to the 'corporate' organizational objectives. However, this may sit uneasily with the professional's sense of responsibility to an individual patient or client. There will never be an easy answer to these dilemmas but professional groups have a particular responsibility to ensure that 'cost–benefit' analysis is never allowed to become all-consuming and dominate all other considerations.

In the previous chapter, mention was made of the welcome Immanuel Kant gave to the Enlightenment, for enabling individuals to escape the 'immaturity' inherent in an, 'inability to use one's understanding without guidance from another'. He was challenging the influence of factors such as emotion and tradition but Kant also stressed the responsibilities this places on us. Drawing attention to the limitations of applying instrumental calculation to every human choice, he urges: 'Act in such a way that you always treat humanity, whether in your own person or in the person of any other, never simply as a means, but always at the same time as an end' (cited in Grayling 2003: 152).

In saying this, Kant recognized the importance of rational thought being grounded in responsible human relationships. However, respecting the uniqueness of others can require responses at an emotional as well as a rational level. This is not to imply that rational dialogue should be abandoned in favour of a vapid sentimentalism but to suggest that the emotional content of health work needs to be properly recognized.

Health care and the role of emotions

The development of rational thinking associated with the Enlightenment was welcomed by many, but one source of objection came from those described as 'Romantics':

> Romantics interpreted the Enlightenment's championship of science as amounting to the claim that scientific development is synonymous with progress itself, which if so would mean that history and human experience can only properly be understood in mechanistic, even deterministic terms. As a way of recoiling from this degree (as they saw it) of rationalism and mechanism, the Romantics asserted instead the primacy of emotion over reason, and accordingly celebrated the subjective, the personal, the visionary and the irrational. They gave a privileged place to moods and passions as sources of insight and as arbiters of truth.
>
> (Grayling 2004: 140–1)

Most people who accept a need for rational, scientific explanations also acknowledge the importance of emotional, subjective experiences. However, difficulties remain in terms of how much weight should be given to each. A lack of attention to emotional aspects has been highlighted by the Bristol Heart Children Action Group, an organization set up by parents of children who died following cardiac surgery at the Bristol Royal Infirmary:

> The medical profession are removed from the needs of the users on an emotional level and because of the very difficult job they do, communication often only stays at a clinical level ... The patient needs to be listened to in whatever form they express themselves ... Gone are the days when the patient needs to be protected by the profession. Far more account should be taken about what patients want and feel they need to know.
>
> (Bristol Heart Children Action Group paper, Kennedy 2001: 292)

In an article arguing the need for the profile of emotional care to be raised in nurse training, Smith (1991) describes the development of the 'nursing process' as having been guided by a desire for nursing to become less 'task-oriented' and more 'person-focused', giving more attention to emotional and psychological aspects of care. However, her own study of nursing students led to the conclusion that this faced an important constraint: 'technical nursing was seen as prestigious and valuable to learning. Indeed, one group described meeting patients' social needs as "not really nursing"' (Smith 1991).

Very early in the history of the NHS, the government minister who oversaw its construction, Aneurin Bevan, appears to have adopted a similar line when facing demands to keep small cottage hospitals open. Urging progress towards developing larger acute hospitals, Bevan's view was expressed bluntly: 'I would rather be kept alive in the efficient if cold altruism of a large hospital than expire in a gush of sympathy in a small one' (Bevan, quoted in Webster 1991).

Faced with the choice, most of us would probably agree. Yet, the contrast between the two environments highlights an important issue about the emotional content of health care work. Specifically, there is a risk of counter-posing 'reason' and 'emotion' in a way that implies professionals bring a rational, scientific knowledge base, in contrast to irrational and emotional evidence relied upon by patients.

This problem is reflected in a study by James (1992), in which a former hospital nurse is interviewed about her current work in a hospice. The nurse describes some of the adjustments needed in moving between the two institutional environments: 'If you're sitting on someone's bed talking, you keep looking round, expecting someone to tell you to do something' (James 1992). The implication being that 'doing something' involves a physical task and thus talking with a patient is relegated in importance to more technical activities. A contrast between technical and emotional tasks arises in many contexts and can be associated with other features of society, notably traditional gender roles. The relationship between the two, and the status each is accorded, is particularly important in health care.

An example of scientific versus experiential accounts

As a comparison of technical and emotional (or objective and subjective) accounts, the following provides a series of extracts from two descriptions of the use of streptomycin as an antibiotic for respiratory tuberculosis in the late 1940s. Hugely significant in itself, it also provides the first reported randomized control trial, in which the scientific methods of the laboratory are used to examine the effectiveness of clinical interventions. The first set of extracts comes from a report, published in the British Medical Journal (BMJ) in October 1948, describing the trial. These are followed by a more subjective description of the effects of the same drug. The point to consider is not so much which is the true account, but how they differ and complement each other. It is not the details included in each of the two accounts that matters, but the style and tenor of their approach.

The BMJ article begins by describing the context for the trial: 'In future, conclusions regarding the clinical effect of a new chemotherapeutic agent in tuberculosis could be considered valid only if based on adequately controlled clinical trials.'

There follows a detailed account of how the sample used in the study was constructed. From this sample patients were allocated to one of two groups: some patients were to receive bed rest and streptomycin (Group C) with others having only bed rest (Group S). It was deemed essential that patients were unaware of the group in which they had been placed. The results showed that four of the 55 patients (7 per cent) receiving streptomycin (Group C) died within six months, compared to 14 of the 52 patients (27 per cent) having only bed rest (Group S). The article notes: 'The difference between the two series is statistically significant; the probability of it occurring by chance is less than one in a hundred.' The article refers to the need to take account of more than the data on mortality, in particular:

> changes in the radiological picture, changes in general condition, temperature, weight, sedimentation rate, and bacillary content of the sputum. We have not attempted a numerical evaluation of the relative importance of each of these, and changes in them will be reported in turn ... So far as possible, the analysis in this report will deal with the more readily measurable data only.

A short section describes the 'general condition' of patients:

> At four months after admission the general condition had improved in 40 (73 per cent) of the 55 S patients, compared with 26 (50 per cent) of 52 C patients; only seven (13 per cent) S patients were worse, whereas 10 (19 per cent) C patients had died and another 13 (25 per cent) were worse than on admission. At six months after admission the difference between the two groups was less; in 33 (60 per cent) S patients and in 24 (46 per cent) C patients the general condition was better than on admission: 13 S patients (24 per cent) were worse and four others (7 per cent) had died; 12 C patients (23 per cent) were worse and 14 others (27 per cent) had died.

Details follow of specific clinical measures, before mention is made of possible toxic side effects of the drug:

> By far the most important toxic effect was the damage to the vestibular apparatus. Giddiness was a frequent first symptom; it was noticed by 36 of the 55 patients, and first appeared on sitting up in bed or turning the head suddenly. It appeared usually in the fourth or fifth week of therapy, and persisted for periods varying from one week to several months ... It is highly desirable that standard tests be adopted for assessment of vestibular dysfunction.

Here again, the emphasis is put upon establishing a standardized, more objective measure, before a brief mention is made of other effects:

> Many patients suffered from nausea and vomiting, symptoms which were often relieved by antihistamine therapy. Albuminuria and casts in urine, raised blood urea, pruritus and urticarial rash, eosinophilia, 'yellow vision' after injection, and circumoral numbness are among other transient effects reported. All subsided spontaneously – i.e., without stopping treatment.
>
> (British Medical Journal 1948)

Throughout, the style is one of detached, objective, scientific enquiry. Only that which is quantifiable receives detailed attention. The objective is to provide a clear and authoritative assessment of the effect of streptomycin upon clinically measurable symptoms.

Now consider the following extracts, taken from the writings of the author George Orwell. Orwell, whose best-known work includes the novels *1984* and *Animal Farm*, may well have contracted tuberculosis when travelling in the 1920s for his book, *Down and Out in Paris and London*. It was not, however, diagnosed until much later, and he was unwell by the time he and his wife adopted a three-week-old boy, Richard, in 1944. Orwell's wife died during surgery in the following year, by which time his own health was deteriorating. During the course of the MRC streptomycin trials, Orwell was told of the drug by his thoracic surgeon, Bruce Dick. In February 1948 Orwell wrote to his friend David Astor seeking a 'rare favour', asking for assistance in getting the drug from America (Crick 1980: 537). A supply of the drug was obtained and by March 1948, Orwell was writing from his hospital bed in Lanarkshire to Julian Symons, a fellow writer.

> I thought you'd like to hear that I am getting a lot better. I have been having the streptomycin for about a month, and evidently it is doing its stuff. I haven't gained much weight, but I am much better in every other way, and longing to get up, which of course they won't let me do for ages yet.
>
> (Orwell and Angus 1970: 461)

However, within a month, writing again to Symons, Orwell reported problems:

> I am a lot better, but I had a bad fortnight with the secondary effects of the streptomycin. I suppose with all these drugs it's rather a case of sinking the ship to get rid of the rats. However, they've stopped the strepto now and evidently it has done its stuff. I am still fearfully weak and thin, but they seem pleased with my case and I think I may get out some time during the summer.
>
> (Orwell and Angus 1970: 472)

Orwell provides a retrospective account of his experience of streptomycin in his final notebook, in an entry dated 24 March 1949. A year after first being treated with the drug, he describes the secondary symptoms it produced:

> Streptomycin was then almost a new drug and had never been used at that hospital before. The symptoms in my case were quite different from those described in the American medical journal in which we read the subject up beforehand.
>
> At first, though the streptomycin seemed to produce an almost immediate improvement in my health, there were no secondary symptoms, except that a sort of discolouration appeared at the base of my fingers and toe nails. Then my face became noticeably redder and the skin had a tendency to flake off, and

a sort of rash appeared all over my body, especially down my back. There was no itching associated with this. After about 3 weeks I got a severe sore throat, which did not go away and was not affected by sucking penicillin lozenges. It was very painful to swallow and I had to have a special diet for some weeks. There was now ulceration with blisters in my throat and in the insides of my cheeks, and the blood kept coming up into little blisters on my lips. At night these burst and bled considerably, so that in the morning my lips were always stuck together with blood and I had to bathe them before I could open my mouth. Meanwhile my nails had disintegrated at the roots and the disintegration grew, as it were, up the nail, new nails forming beneath meanwhile. My hair began to come out, and one or two patches of quite white hair appeared at the back (previously it was only speckled with grey).

After 50 days the streptomycin, which had been injected at the rate of 1 gramme a day, was discontinued. The lips etc. healed almost immediately and the rash went away, though not quite so promptly. My hair stopped coming out and went back to its normal colour, though I think with more grey in it than before. The old nails ended by dropping out altogether, and some months after leaving hospital I only had ragged tips, which kept splitting, to the new nails. Some of the toenails did not drop out. Even now my nails are not normal. They are much more corrugated than before, and a great deal thinner, with a constant tendency to split if I do not keep them very short.

(Quoted in Crick 1980: 539–40)

Writing to one of his oldest friends, Richard Rees, on 8 April 1949, Orwell reveals a continuing decline in spite of the earlier course of streptomycin:

I've had the sanatorium cable the magazines to which I had promised articles saying I am unfit to do any work, which is the truth. Don't depress the others too much with this, but the fact is I am in a bad way at present. They are going to try streptomycin again, which I had previously urged them to do and which Mr Dick thought might be a good idea. They had been afraid of it because of the secondary effects, but they now say they can offset these to some extent and in any case they can always stop if the results are too bad. *If* things go badly – of course we'll hope they won't, but one must be prepared for the worst – I'll ask you to bring little Richard to see me before I get too frightening in appearance. I think it would upset you less than it would Avril [Orwell's sister], and there may be business deals to talk over as well. If the stuff works, as it seemed to do last time, I shall take care this time to keep the improvement by leading an invalid life for the rest of the year.

(In Orwell and Angus 1970: 549)

George Orwell died nine months later, at the age of 46.

Working with emotions

These accounts of the effects of streptomycin reveal different types of information, and the real challenge lies in how to incorporate objective and subjective forms of knowledge to deepen understanding. Too much emphasis on one over the other provides a partial and limited perspective. Although there can be a tendency to put more reliance on technical measurements and skills, much of the work of health professionals involves a kind of work that has been described as 'emotional labour' (Hochschild 1983), in which feelings and emotions are suppressed as part of a formal role, thereby creating for others the appearance and image that the institutional context requires. Hochschild developed the idea from research into the handling of emotions by airline cabin staff, but the concept of emotional labour has been applied in health care settings by others. Among these Nicky James explains: 'I define emotional labour as the labour involved in dealing with other people's feelings, a core component of which is the regulation of emotions ... Emotional labour facilitates and regulates the expression of emotion in the public domain' (James 1989: 15).

A related concept is that of 'sentimental work', defined by Strauss *et al.* as, 'any work where the object being worked on is alive and sentient' (Strauss *et al.* 1982: 254).

Emotions matter, not only because they cause us to have different feelings but because these, in turn, can influence the way we think and make decisions. While it remains hugely important to maintain the Enlightenment tradition of scientific analysis and rational thought, this cannot displace entirely more subjective and experiential accounts. As will be discussed in Chapter 5, the balance between reason and emotion assumes special significance within the patient–professional relationship. It is also important, in this context, to consider the role of traditional knowledge and beliefs.

Health and the role of traditional beliefs

Just as our health can be a matter of intense emotional concern, so too it can be subject to long-standing, traditional ideas and beliefs. The role of lay accounts and explanations for illness prompted several pieces of sociological research in the 1980s and 1990s, an early example of which was based on interviews with 46 middle-aged, working-class women in Scotland (Blaxter 1983). When asked about factors they saw as contributing to disease and ill-health, the women responded with a wide range including infection and the environment, heredity, individual susceptibility, stress and psychological explanations, ageing, among others.

Blaxter noted that comments made by the women reflected different ways of identifying the cause of illness, particularly between the immediate cause of a disease and its earlier antecedents or origins. She uses the example of influenza to illustrate how its cause may be defined in terms of infection by a virus but the outcome will also be determined by the state of the immune system. This, in turn, will be the result of a host of other factors.

The fact that many diseases have multiple 'causes' is developed by Blaxter to consider how lay and scientific accounts may differ in their focus:

> Ideas about cause were a very important component of the models of disease held by this particular social group. Their 'preferred' categories of cause can be shown to be a product of their particular social situation. Their general models of causal process, painstakingly derived from their own experience as they saw it, were often scientifically wrong in detail, but were not in principle unscientific.
>
> (Blaxter 1983: 68)

In other words, simple mono-causal explanations may identify the specific agent that was the immediate cause of a disease but this effect will have been determined by many other influences. It was to these that many of the women referred when they identified the causes of disease. Blaxter's study indicates the need to consider the meaning of lay accounts carefully. It is also worth bearing in mind that lay knowledge itself can be the product of previous expert knowledge. For instance, during the 1970s and 1980s parents of newborn babies were advised by health professionals to place them to sleep on their fronts to reduce the risk of cot deaths. The rationale was that if a baby regurgitated milk, it was less likely to choke than if it was laying on its back. Research evidence began to emerge that questioned this view and in October 1991 the Chief Medical Officer convened an expert group to review all that was available, and it concluded that babies placed on their backs had lower risk of cot death. In fact, this had been the advice since 1989 given by professionals in Bristol, where rates had fallen.

> As a result from December 1991 the Department of Health and the media ran a campaign to educate parents (the Back to Sleep campaign). Cot deaths have halved in the years since the campaign. This is an example of rapid, active learning in the NHS which led to the saving of over 3,000 babies' lives in the six years up to 1998.
>
> (Department of Health 2000: 32)

By the early 1990s, many new parents would have been babies themselves in the 1970s. Their own parents would presumably have received the opposite advice to that which they were receiving. It seems reasonable to assume that in some cases this may have created confusion. The 'lay knowledge' possessed by the babies' grandparents may now be judged wrong, but originally came from the very same source as today's expert view.

Another important aspect of lay knowledge about health is the way in which 'health' itself is understood, an aspect explored in a study conducted around the same time as Blaxter's. This study used intensive, open-ended interviews with 70 people aged 60 and over living in Aberdeen, Scotland, plus more structured interviews with a random sample of the same age group (Williams, 1983). Williams suggests three main dimensions along which health was understood. The first was the absence of illness and disease; this was generally defined in terms of restrictions on normal activities. Second, health was seen as strength, with its opposite being weakness. People who had a disease would sometimes describe themselves as healthy, defining this as a constitutional characteristic. Others might be seen as unhealthy because of vulnerability and susceptibility to illness and infection. Notions of energy and exhaustion were closely connected with this idea.

Third, Williams discusses health as functional fitness:

> for my informants, the existence of weaknesses in their constitution did not on its own imply that they were unfit for their normal activities. This was most clearly seen in cases where a constitutional weakness existed unaccompanied by current disabling disease. In such cases the sufferer might indeed feel vulnerable; but vulnerability on its own, unaccompanied by a recognized disease, was felt as inadequate grounds for excusing oneself from normal social obligations.
>
> (Williams 1983: 193)

One woman with hypertension, for example, felt torn between accepting invitations to social events that she did not really want to go to and that might irritate her, or rejecting them in spite of having a condition that was 'not an illness' (Williams 1983: 193). Medicine plays an important role in providing a clinical diagnosis but this may not always determine how others judge these conditions. Diagnosis of a clinical condition does not necessarily mean it is regarded as a 'real' illness. This is an issue developed by Jocelyn Cornwell, whose work provides a focus for the remainder of this section.

Defining 'health problems'

Cornwell's study involved a detailed investigation into the lives of 24 people, 15 women and nine men, living in East London:

> Its chief concern is with their commonsense ideas and theories about health, illness, and health services, but it is based on the assumption that if we are to understand the significance they attach to this, as to any areas of their lives, then we have to consider its place in the context of their lives as a whole.
>
> (Cornwell 1984: 1)

Habermas and rationality

Before summarizing some of Cornwell's empirical findings, a few remarks should be made about the approach she adopts. This draws upon the work of Jürgen Habermas, former Professor of Philosophy and Sociology at the University of Frankfurt. Habermas has written extensively about the modern world but an aspect relevant for this discussion concerns his development of Weber's ideas on processes of rationalization in modern society. Weber discussed different forms of rationality but regarded the process of rationalization as one that led increasingly to the dominance of 'formal rationality'. He went so far as to describe this as the 'iron cage of rationalisation', reflecting concern that factors other than scientific and technological considerations are becoming increasingly marginalized.

The term 'purposive rationality' is used by Habermas to describe processes in modern society akin to what Weber described as *Zweckrationalitat*, or formal rationality. But Habermas was not convinced that this had the overbearing dominance suggested by Weber. This dominance is achieved, for Habermas, not in all spheres of life but in those characterized by systems: the economic system; political system; social system; and so on. This 'system world' is contrasted by Habermas with what he refers to as a 'lifeworld', in which a wider range of cultural practices and attitudes dominate. The way in which Habermas defines the lifeworld can appear a little impenetrable but essentially it can be thought of as comprising 'background knowledge' rather than formal, scientific knowledge. It represents the assumptions, beliefs, attitudes that we hold; ways of thinking that are tacit rather than explicit. It is our 'common sense'.

The distinction between the 'lifeworld and 'system world' is paralleled by another concerning the basis on which social action is justified, or legitimized. Habermas contrasts 'traditional legitimation', which is drawn from religious or moral belief systems and is primarily normative, with 'modern legitimations', requiring scientific and technical knowledge. Whereas the former is grounded in the values people hold, the latter is founded upon analytic or empirical knowledge.

Cornwell's approach

The distinction between traditional and modern legitimation provides Cornwell with a means of understanding the wider role that scientific and medical knowledge comes to play:

> 'Rationalization' is the process that takes place when social life is transformed by traditional legitimations being overturned and replaced by modern ones ... traditional legitimations are undermined and they lose their cogency – people lose faith in them – in the face of modern scientific and technical forms of argument which eventually replace them. Medicalization as used in this study is the specific form which rationalization takes in the area of health and illness. Medicalization 'from above' describes the changes in the Western view of mind and body that have occurred with the development of scientific medicine. Medicalization 'from below' describes the changes in social life and social relations that create a readiness on the part of sub-cultures and the individuals who belong to them to accept modern (in this case, medical) legitimations for health and illness where once they accepted traditional (common sense and moralistic) legitimations.
>
> (Cornwell 1984: 119–20)

Cornwell is careful to acknowledge the capacity of traditional ideas to retain their influence. She is not suggesting that medicalization represents the absolute domination of scientific explanations. Instead:

It states the dominant tendency in our culture, which is towards modern scientific and technical forms of legitimation, without implying that the process will necessarily be carried through everywhere and in all social groups, at the same pace or at the same time. The rate of progress of medicalization depends upon the state of readiness of sub-cultures to allow it to take place, and on their state of awareness and knowledge of scientific achievements.

(Cornwell 1984: 120)

Cornwell develops this approach to reflect on comments made by those who were interviewed in the study, describing personal experiences of illness:

The onus on the person giving the account was to that of proving that the illness was 'real' and that it was therefore legitimate for them – or whoever was involved – to be a patient. The basic requirement was that they should be able to prove the 'otherness' of the illness, i.e., prove that it was a recognisable and separate entity which had 'happened' to the person and not something for which they were personally responsible.

(pp. 129–30)

Cornwell suggests that it is in situations such as this that 'common sense' and 'medical' legitimations interact:

The most conclusive proof of the 'reality' of an illness the person could offer was a medical diagnosis. The scientific discourse of medicine thus provided the major solution to the moral difficulties of illness; once there was a recognisably medical diagnosis the question of individual responsibility and culpability were no longer relevant.

(p. 130)

Categorizing health problems

Cornwell's approach is important because of the recognition it gives to the interaction between lay and medical knowledge. This is demonstrated in a description of three different ways in which health problems were differentiated by respondents in the study.

The first is described as 'normal' illness, and includes infectious diseases that were either expected in childhood, or common among adults but not severe. These were regarded as being amenable to medical treatment, which was normally effective. Illnesses of this kind were distinguished from 'real' illness, which included more serious, disabling and possibly life-threatening illness, such as cancer and coronary heart disease. They are generally severe, in many cases having a poor prognosis, being 'just within or just beyond the province of successful medical treatment' (Cornwell 1984: 130).

Third, were 'health problems which are not illness'. From the point of view of the relationship between medical and traditional forms of knowledge these can be the most important. With the rising incidence of chronic disease, it is noteworthy that 'health problems which are not illness' tended to be associated with natural processes, such as ageing and the reproductive cycle, and problems thought to stem from the person's nature or personality: 'The common feature of this category of problems is that they are thought not to be amenable to medical treatment' (Cornwell 1984: 131).

Cornwell explains:

> Health problems that are regarded as a natural part of growing old are: rheumatism; arthritis; digestive disorders; varicose veins; palpitations; and feeling the cold, as well as loss of hearing and vision. The problems that menstruation and the menopause account for are many and various: they include abdominal pain; sickness; nausea; palpitations; hot flushes; blood loss; changes in weight; faintness and dizziness; depression and other mood changes; and changes in the condition and texture of the hair.
>
> (Cornwell 1984: 131)

For these conditions, people would be expected to 'cope', perhaps through self-treatment, with a stronger likelihood of them being considered responsible for the progress of the condition. For example, one interviewee mentioned that his nephew had eczema as a child, going on to say:

> It's a disease, isn't it? And I don't think they really know how it occurs or anything like that. And it's definitely not through dirt because ... my sister's house is as clean if not cleaner than most people's ... And it wasn't through the food because she's a real good cook.
>
> (Cornwell 1984: 132)

The identification of something as a 'disease' is used to establish the causes as being 'external'. Medicine may not understand how it is caused, but it is sufficient to suggest that the individual – and in this case his parents – are not responsible. In addition to the diagnostic label confirming that the symptoms are genuine, it also serves to attribute the cause of the disease to factors beyond the victim's control. In this sense, diagnosis can provide almost a moral role, influencing the attribution of responsibility.

Illness and its social setting

Cornwell's approach helps us think about how and why symptoms are seen as significant or not. These assessments are made in specific contexts, which help define what is regarded as normal or out of the ordinary. Other sociological and anthropological work points to the role our social milieu plays in determining these responses. If nearly everyone around us has the same condition, then it ceases to have the relatively distinctive character typically associated with illness.

In an article, 'Culture and symptoms: an analysis of patients' presenting complaints', the American sociologist Irving Zola describes studies going back to the 1950s that explore these issues. In one, Margaret Clark found diarrhoea, sweating and coughing to be everyday experiences among many Mexican-Americans in the South-western United States, and in another Richard Blum found trachoma (a contagious disease of the eye causing inflammation) almost universal among some Greeks. Both studies suggested that where conditions affected almost everyone, they received little attention. They are judged as being 'normal' rather than 'deviant' (Zola 1975).

Another study from the 1950s, conducted in the United States, found that although lower back pain was quite common among 'lower-class' women it was not regarded as indicative of any underlying disorder or disease. Because it was so ubiquitous it was expected and therefore seen as part of the normal human condition. (Koos 1954, cited in Zola 1972). An appreciation of the role others play in shaping our own perceptions of what is normal, is developed by the American sociologist, Eliot Freidson, to consider the role of 'lay referral networks'. Freidson saw lay referral networks as part of a 'lay referral structure', itself an element in a much larger process: 'The whole process of seeking help involves a network of potential consultants, from the intimate and informal confines of the nuclear family through successively more select, distant and authoritative laymen, until the "professional" is reached' (Freidson 1960).

These are themes developed in later chapters: here some general observations on the relationships between science, values, emotion and tradition provide a conclusion to this chapter.

Relationships between science, values, emotion and tradition

Science has made an enormous contribution to human progress. Without the knowledge it has developed, many more deaths and far more suffering would occur. However, medical science cannot supply answers to all questions, and even where scientific explanations are available, they may only provide a partial account. Intense emotions, of love, fear, joy or anxiety, may be described scientifically in terms of various neurotransmitters but chemical changes in the brain do not explain the experience of feeling these emotions. What is more, scientific conclusions have sometimes been proven wrong, and others have brought unanticipated problems.

Modern medicine and health care have brought real benefits but the knowledge it relies on can be tentative, uncertain, partial and sometimes wrong. It should not surprise us that the view of scientific experts is not always embraced by others. Acknowledging this is an important element in establishing a relationship between patients and professionals capable of accommodating different perspectives. For it cannot be assumed that the ultimate objective must always be to ensure the expert, scientific view prevails.

To reiterate a point made earlier, this is not to reduce all problems to determination by feeling and emotion. It is to recognize that scientific assessments can themselves incorporate assumptions that need to be questioned. This is illustrated in remarks made by a public health official in the United States, after working with local people to investigate the health consequences of pollution in the neighbourhood of Love Canal.

The neighbourhood, in New York State, was one of family housing, built on the site of a former waste disposal site where over 20,000 tons of toxic chemicals had been dumped in the 1940s. When residents complained of odours and 'substances' coming to the surface no action was taken, despite the identification of toxic residues. The view was taken that these posed no significant risk to health.

Eventually, with media attention in the 1970s bringing the issue to public attention, the New York state commissioner for health ordered that the exposed chemicals be removed. In 1978, the then US President, Jimmy Carter, declared a federal emergency, providing funds to relocate over two hundred families.

Having worked with local residents, one public health official reflected on the effect of this experience:

> Before Love Canal, I also needed a 95 per cent certainty before I was con-vinced of a result. But seeing this rigorously applied in a situation where the consequences of an error meant that pregnancies were resulting in mis-carriages, stillbirths and children with medical problems, I realized I was making a value judgement . . . whether to make errors on the side of protecting human health or on the side of conserving state resources.
>
> (Quoted in Brown 1995: 97)

This recalls the relationship between 'personal troubles' and 'public issues' that C. Wright Mills identified as central to the sociological imagination. It is a theme developed further in the next chapter, which explores some of the ways that clinical diagnosis has implications for personal and social domains. Discussion on the private and public meanings associated with diagnosis also provides an appropriate context for considering the relationship between patients and pro-fessionals in Chapter 5.

4
Diagnosis, meaning and experience

Sociologically, the importance of a diagnostic label is the status it gives the person to whom it is applied. This is true whether the label describes an illness, a disability, or quite different conditions, such as pregnancy. The status granted by a diagnosis can produce positive benefits, such as access to appropriate treatment, but also potentially negative ones, including the possibility of stigma and discrimination. This chapter considers some of these social meanings and consequences of diagnosis but first, attention is given to the more immediate, personal impact.

The two are intimately connected. The whole approach of this book emphasizes the interconnections between the personal and the social. One cannot be understood without taking account of the other. Nevertheless, sequentially it is useful to begin by looking at diagnosis from a personal perspective, helping to focus attention on relevant aspects for later sections.

Diagnosis is often relatively straightforward. A woman may be uncertain about whether or not she is pregnant, for instance, but once a period has been missed might seek to have this determined with a reasonably high degree of accuracy. Blood tests would be capable of confirming the diagnosis at an even earlier stage, before the woman herself would be aware of more obvious signs. However, confirmation of pregnancy may not eliminate other uncertainties. For a woman aged over 35, for instance, this might prompt further investigative tests, such as amniocentesis, on the grounds of an increased statistical probability of chromosomal abnormalities being present.

Likewise, there are many illnesses where the diagnosis can be relatively easy and uncontroversial. This is not always so. Problems of determining an accurate diagnosis can be particularly evident in areas of chronic illness and mental health. For this reason, the chapter begins by considering the importance of diagnosis for the individual, approaching it in C. Wright Mills' phrase as a 'personal trouble'. This is followed by a section that identifies some of the 'public issues' relating to diagnosis, before describing four approaches to understanding the relationship between the two.

These four approaches differ considerably in their focus, but each seeks to aid understanding of the meaning that can be given to diagnoses, both by the individual and by wider society. Three of the approaches consider how and why 'illness' has become such an important category for explaining human experiences, while the other focuses on some of the negative social consequences that diagnosis can bring, particularly as a source of stigma. When considering each of them, it is worth thinking about the idea that a considerable amount of illness in modern society has its roots in psychosocial factors. Although this theme is not necessarily explicit, it provides an important critique of accounts focusing predominantly upon the physical and biological consequences. Possible psychosocial causes of illness are considered in Chapters 8 and 9 but it is important also to note the relevance of these ideas to debates about the ways in which illness is defined and explained.

Diagnosis as a 'personal trouble'

Diagnosis of a seriously debilitating or life-threatening condition is a profoundly traumatic experience. An important feature of these situations is the means by which information is communicated and shared with the patient and their relatives, something which is considered in a little more detail in Chapter 5. However, even where a diagnosis is not of this type, its impact can be considerable.

To illustrate this, the section begins with a series of extracts taken from an account given by a doctor of the experience of an individual patient, written in 1954. They indicate how, without a diagnosis, individuals can feel uncertain and anxious, and perhaps sensitive to the possibility of being seen by others as malingering rather than genuinely ill (originally published in Balint 1957).

The extracts record parts of a consultation between Michael Balint, a doctor and psychotherapist, and a patient. The patient, Mr U, aged 36, is a skilled workman who overcame disability caused by childhood polio. Married with a family, his youngest child, aged four, has been quite seriously ill. Mr U has also suffered illness since having an accident at work and consequently visits his GP:

> Earlier that year Mr U had an accident at work, after an electrical connection had been interfered with, causing him to receive a very severe shock. After being unconscious for about fifteen minutes he revived and was examined by a doctor. Mr U had later gone to see his own doctor, complaining of pains in his chest, back, right leg, and right hand. He linked this with the electric shock, and although there was no evidence of organic damage, he was referred to a specialist.

An issue here is that of attribution – how we explain the cause of an experience. The patient is relating his recently developed pains to a significant, perhaps life-threatening, event that occurred shortly before these emerged. The doctor does not believe there is any organic, or physical, damage but the chronological sequence provides the patient with some grounds for his reasoning. It undoubtedly provokes his anxiety, the reason for which a hospital referral is made. After seeing the specialist, Mr U returns to his GP who recounts:

The letter to me from the hospital said that they could not find anything, and that 'we would like the patient to be seen by our psychiatrist'. I told him that nothing wrong had been found, and he said that was funny because his pains were much worse. He said, 'They seem to think I am imagining things – I know what I have got.' After talking a few minutes in a very pleasant manner, he said he thought the hospital might have made a mistake. He is definitely ill, and would like to know what condition he could have causing all these pains. 'What does the book say about it?'

(p. 136)

Michael Balint comments:

He came to his old trusted friend, the family doctor, prompted by pains, anxieties, fears but otherwise in a trusting and friendly mood, hoping for help, understanding, and sympathy. It is true that he received a fair amount of all of them, but was then put through the mill of a routine hospital examination, almost certainly with a number of white-coated strangers firing searching questions at him. Perhaps he did, perhaps he did not, realize that everybody was getting more and more concerned about a possible claim for compensation, or to use a more fashionable term, about a compensation neurosis, and trying their best to prevent him sliding into it. What he certainly did realize, however, was that all the doctors were at pains to convince him that *there was nothing wrong with him, i.e. they were rejecting his proposition.* When he came back to his doctor with the hospital report, the previous trusting, friendly attitude had been badly shaken, the model patient had turned into a disappointed, suspicious, mistrustful man.

(p. 137)

Michael Balint notes that the experience of the hospital examination changed the relationship between the patient and the doctor, which in this particular case had been very good. His account continues:

Only when the patient suspected that the doctors would somehow reject his 'propositions', i.e. either did not understand his illness, or, still worse, did not care to understand it, did the relationship suffer. The patient started feeling – dimly at first – that perhaps the doctors were no longer on his side, that possibly they were actually against him. The hitherto model patient was thus forced first into an argument with his doctor, an argument which might later develop into a major battle. Yet we should not forget that despite this strain and suspicion the patient is still frightened and lost, desperately in need of help. His chief problem which he cannot solve without help, is: what is his illness, the thing that has caused his pains and frightens him? In his own words, 'What does the book say?'

I wish to emphasize here that nearly always this is the chief and most immediate problem; *the request for a name for the illness, for a diagnosis.* It is only in the second instance that the patient asks for therapy, i.e. what can be done to alleviate his sufferings on the one hand, and the restrictions and deprivations caused by the illness, on the other.

Not paying attention to this order of importance is the cause of a very frequent form of irritation and of bitter disappointment in the doctor–patient relationship.

(pp. 137–8)

The desire for a diagnosis, as an authoritative judgement of a condition, can run into difficulties where the nature of a complaint is complex and uncertain. A definitive diagnosis can be difficult to make, or more than one possible explanation may present itself. Some examples of this are found in a report of three fairly small Australian studies of women with a chronic illness, which describe accounts of women's responses to the diagnosis of illness (Kralik, Brown and Koch 2001). Unsurprisingly, women typically recounted the receipt of a diagnosis negatively, but despite this recalled how: 'it was important for them to know the illness had a name. A diagnosis meant that the illness was validated by medical science and was then perceived by others to be real' (Kralik, Brown and Koch 2001: 595).

One woman described her feelings when told that a blood test had revealed an abnormality:

. . . at last a bloody test was showing something was going on, and it was not in my head, so worried or not, I was relieved to finally be proved I was telling the truth, and I have to say that had they even given me a diagnoses of something really bad and terminal, I was just glad at that time, that now, I knew I was right, and I was not making this all up. Now it was up to them.

(Kralik, Brown and Koch 2001: 598)

In many circumstances, 'a medical diagnosis also meant the possibility of treatment and cure' but this was not always the case. Even here, though, knowing what was causing the symptoms could still be desired: 'Upon diagnosis I actually felt relief mixed with fear. Relieved because the problem had a name, fearful because there is no cure and no known cause' (Kralik, Brown and Koch 2001: 598)

Other women, those still awaiting a diagnosis: 'lived day to day with uncertainty and disrupted self-identity. As health professionals we should not underestimate the desire for a medical diagnostic label' (Kralik, Brown and Koch 2001: 595).

Similar experiences are described by Lesley Cooper in a study of ten people suffering from Myalgic Encephalomyelitis (ME), many of whom described difficult encounters with doctors who did not recognize the symptoms as a diagnosable disease (Cooper 1997).

The role a diagnosis can play is not solely a consequence of what it may mean for an individual in terms of the future. It can also have a major impact on how an individual understands and explains their experiences, to others as well as to themselves. One important emotional consequence of a clinical diagnosis is that it provides a socially acceptable explanation for behaviour that might otherwise be viewed more negatively. It can provide a legitimate reason for withdrawing from normal social obligations. This is one reason why diagnoses are simultaneously 'personal troubles' and 'public issues'.

Diagnosis as a 'public issue'

One way that diagnoses become a public issue is the justification they may provide for being unable to work. This may sometimes be challenged, as suggested in this news report:

> According to a report by the health insurance company, Norwich Union, GPs suspected that of the 9 million sick notes requested every year, one in five was invalid. Other estimates suggest that more than a third of sick notes issued each year might be bogus.
>
> The British Medical Association said the report backed its efforts to shift the job of issuing sick notes to company occupational health departments.
>
> (*Financial Times* 28.04.04)

According to surveys by the Confederation of British Industry (CBI) and the Chartered Institute of Personnel and Development (CIPD), short-term sickness accounts for 80 per cent of absences, with minor illnesses such as colds, stomach upsets and headaches the most common cause. However, long-term sickness accounts for 40 per cent of total working days lost (Barham and Leonard 2002).

Between 1980–1 and 1995–6 the total days of medically-certified incapacity due to sickness and invalidity rose from 345,300,000 to 874,900,000 (DSS statistics), an enormous increase. Put into perspective, the highest number of working days ever lost in any year through industrial action – in 1926, the year of the General Strike – was 162,233,000. By 1999 the total was a mere 242,000.

With much of this sickness accounted for by long-term sickness, absence from work has actually stayed fairly constant, at around 3.2 per cent. In contrast, according to the General Household Survey, a large-scale representative survey conducted each year, the proportion of British adults with a limiting long-term illness rose from 21 per cent in 1972 to 35 per cent in 2000 (Bartley, Sacker and Clarke 2004). This proportion represents those who describe themselves in this way, and does not require any independent assessment. The 2001 census for England and Wales records 9,484,856 people describing themselves as having a limiting, long-term illness, and 4,797,343 who described their general health as 'not good'. Of these totals, 2,464,717 adults were unable to be in employment because of permanent sickness or disability.

Rising levels of long-term sickness in the 1980s and 1990s were blamed by some Labour politicians on an alleged strategy by the former Conservative government to remove people from the unemployment statistics. Speaking in April 2004, the New Labour government's work and pensions minister, Des Browne, expressed concern about a 'culture of worklessness' existing in many inner-city areas:

> Mr Browne said the legacy of the Conservatives' drive to push people off the jobless roll on to sickness-related benefits was partly to blame. Once people have claimed sickness-related benefits for more than a year, their chances of going back to work decline steeply … One million of those on incapacity benefit say they would like a job, according to ministry research.
>
> (*Guardian* 01.04.04)

Recent years have seen a levelling off of the number of people entitled to receive incapacity benefit (IB), paid to people medically assessed as being incapable of work. For example, 1,486,200 people under pension age received IB in early 2004, a small decline from 1,559,000 in early 1995. The figure that tends to be quoted in the media and by politicians is the 2.7 million claimants (not all of whom are successful or receive the benefit payment).

However, two features of this development should be noted. First, a very limited range of conditions account for the vast majority of claims. Of the 2004 total of around one and a half million, 813,500 (54 per cent) received the benefit because of just two conditions, mental and behavioural disorders, and diseases of the musculo-skeletal system and the connective tissue (DWP Statistics 2004). Second, the proportion who have received the benefit for five years and more has increased, from 46 per cent in 2000 to 51 per cent in 2003 (Hansard, Written Answers for 15 June 2004). A national survey of incapacity benefit claimants found 64 per cent saying their condition had affected their ability to do paid work for over five years. Ninety per cent anticipated that their conditions would last for at least another year (Loumidis *et al.* 2000: 18).

David Willetts, the shadow work and pensions secretary at the time of writing, now levels the same accusation against the government as was made of the Conservatives: using the category of 'incapacity' to conceal unemployment:

> As the number of people officially unemployed falls, so the number of people on incapacity benefit rises. Gordon Brown isn't really getting people off welfare and into work. He's not getting them off welfare, he's moving them from one benefit to another. This is yet more evidence that when Gordon Brown is celebrating apparent reductions in unemployment, his guilty secret is that he's got more and more people dependent on disability benefits.
>
> (*Daily Telegraph* 28.06.04)

Party political disputes of this kind may throw little light on the problem but they illustrate how criteria for diagnosis can become a high-profile public issue. This becomes especially pertinent for conditions that might be attributable to workplace factors but can prove difficult to diagnose. In one account of Repetitive Strain Injury, or Upper Limb Disorder, which questions the existence of the condition, consultant hand surgeon J. Campbell Semple notes an apparent paradox that reductions in the physical effort required at the workplace is accompanied by increasing numbers of claims for disability (Campbell Semple 1991).

Noting that similar observations have been made in relation to lower back pain in modern society, Semple argues: 'It is therefore important that orthopaedic surgeons clarify their views, try to define what is definable, and attempt to explain, by experiment or rationalisation, that which remains uncertain' (Campbell Semple 1991: 536).

After briefly commenting on a number of recognized pathologies, including tenosynovitis and carpal tunnel syndrome, Semple goes on to consider cases in which no such identifiable pathology exists:

> Where there are no physical signs, what is the diagnosis for work-related discomfort? There may be no diagnosable condition: we all experience inde-terminate aches and pains in the upper limb from time to time. We may well be doing a severe disservice to our patients, and to society, when we strive too hard to categorise every ache or pain into a disease entity or syndrome. A caring doctor may often treat his patient most effectively by confident reas-surance that there is no significant pathology.
>
> (Campbell Semple 1991: 537)

Semple objects to the adoption of 'easy acronyms', such as RSI, by the media and at the workplace, 'despite criticism by authoritative medical organisations' (537). Failure to establish any discernible pathological condition leads Semple to the conclusion that other factors have prompted the rising number of complaints:

> If many people are really suffering the consequences of modern working conditions, then the pathological processes should be defined, the cause dis-covered and the matter resolved by prevention ... If it is true that the chronic use of a keyboard, or jointing chickens all day, actually causes disease or injury to the upper limb, then it should be an easy matter to prove it, but at present there is little positive evidence. Common sense suggests that the present epi-demic of RSI is more likely to be a product of preconceived disability in the workplace, with its opportunity for compensation claims, rather than a widespread 'industrial' injury or disease.
>
> (Campbell Semple 1991: 537)

A very different approach to understanding RSI is provided by Hilary Arksey, who describes unsuccessful attempts to have the condition recognized as a pre-scribed industrial disease (Arksey 1994).

Matters of this kind are significant personal troubles as well as being public issues. So how might the relationship between the two be understood? To suggest some frameworks for thinking about this, the following describes four different approaches. These are not presented as separate or necessarily rival, but simply as different ways of understanding how the personal experience of illness relates to the social circumstances in which it arises.

The first approach considers illness, not in terms of specific characteristics, but in the light of a more general quality: that it represents a deviation from 'normality'. In this sense, it can be described as a form of deviance, an approach particularly associated with the American sociologist, Talcott Parsons. Parsons was interested in trying to understand how society deals with deviance, including illness, and although much of his writing was rather theoretical, he provides an important perspective for thinking about ways in which the personal and the social are related.

One social consequence of receiving certain diagnostic labels is that some can be stigmatizing, perceived negatively by others. A sociologist who has made a significant contribution to thinking about stigma is Erving Goffman, whose work is referred to in the second section below, which includes examples drawn from physical and mental illness. The concept of stigma, and considering why it may arise in particular situations, offers another useful perspective for thinking about the relationship between personal troubles and public issues.

An important line of argument advanced by several writers over several years is the claim that medical diagnosis has been used increasingly to define problems that are not properly within its remit. This is often associated with the notion of 'medicalization', defined as: 'the increasing attachment of medical labels to behaviour regarded as socially or morally undesirable' (Abercrombie, Hall and Turner 1984: 132).

The third section considers some of these arguments, drawing on the work of two writers, the sociologist Irving Zola and a more general critic of modern, industrial society, Ivan Illich. Moving from the role of professional authority, the fourth section considers the part increasingly played by commercial interests in shaping responses to human problems that become defined as illnesses.

Although presenting alternative ways of conceiving the relationship between personal and public issues in diagnoses, there is a common strand that runs through the four approaches. This is the question of how we deal with experiences and behaviours that differ from the normal and typical, and which are capable of being explained by the application of a clinical diagnosis.

Illness and deviance: Talcott Parsons

When we think of behaviour or performance that is normal we might use words such as typical, usual, common or regular. These words need not imply any judgement about the worth of that behaviour but simply recognize it as what might be anticipated. Sometimes behaviour, performance and experiences deviate from the expected. In everyday conversation the word 'deviant' can possess negative or undesirable connotations, but sociologically we can speak of deviance simply as behaviour that breaches commonly accepted norms.

One sociologist who took this approach was the American Talcott Parsons, whose work was influential for many years, although less so today. Nevertheless, concepts he introduced, such as the 'sick role', referred to in the next chapter, have entered a much wider literature, more than justifying his inclusion here.

Central to Parsons' thinking was the concept of a 'social system'. One of his great interests was in how equilibrium was achieved and maintained: what, in essence, makes social order possible? What keeps society functioning? Because of this focus, the school of sociology to which Parsons is associated is often described as 'functionalism' (or 'structural-functionalism'):

> If 'society' is indeed a system in dynamic equilibrium, if it is stable and orderly in this sense, to this extent, then the key question is why this is so. And the standard answer, which defines the functionalist approach to society, is that the equilibrium of the whole derives from the operation of its parts: each part of the social system, each particular social institution, 'functions' in a way that, given how all the other institutions are 'functioning', contributes to the persistence of the whole.
>
> (Barnes 1995: 38)

The analogy might be drawn with a biological system, in which homeostatic mechanisms operate to bring the body into equilibrium. Breathing may become deeper when more oxygen is required, or the heart may pump faster when blood is needed in the muscles. Individual parts of the body are understood in terms of the needs of the system. This, in essence, is how functionalists such as Talcott Parsons seek to explain much of human social behaviour.

So, how can this kind of explanation for human behaviour have anything to say about health and illness? According to Parsons:

> The problem of health is intimately involved in the functional prerequisites of the social system ... Certainly by almost any definition health is included in the functional needs of the individual member of the society ... from the point of view of the functioning of the social system, too low a general level of health, too high an incidence of illness, is dysfunctional: this is in the first instance because illness incapacitates the effective performance of social roles.
>
> (Parsons 1951, cited in Scambler 2002: 14)

For Parsons, illness could be understood as a form of deviance because it prevented those affected from carrying out their normal social roles and responsibilities. His interest was in how a social system responded to deviance of this kind, however, it is worth staying with his description of illness as deviance at this stage in the argument.

Psychological influences on illness

Although a sociologist, Parsons was also interested in psychoanalysis, from which he drew an emphasis upon the unconscious as a source of motivation. The concept of the unconscious has been a controversial one, not least because of the inherent difficulties in observing and studying its functioning. That said, few would dispute the idea that some mental activity occurs of which we are not fully conscious. The

Austrian psychoanalyst, Sigmund Freud, regarded the unconscious as not only the source of our primitive drives but also the repository for past experiences, especially those with strong emotional elements that we repress from our conscious thinking.

The influence of psychoanalytic thinking on Parsons' view of illness can be seen in the way he stresses the interrelationship between psychological and physical factors. Because of this relationship, he suspected that there was likely to be an ever expanding range of sicknesses in situations where individuals experienced problems in coping with social involvement and interaction: 'By their very nature, societies constantly reproduce sickness, and so to speak, invent new categories of sickness to correspond with new strains in the structure of social relations' (Parsons in Turner 1986, cited in Boswell 1992: 173).

It is important to remember that Parsons' principle interest was in understanding social order and the functioning of social systems. Some forms of sickness could thus be viewed as a means of managing the problems people faced in coping with modern life. Parsons consequently became interested in an approach known as psychosomatic medicine, which emphasized the role of the practitioner in combining scientific knowledge and emotional understanding.

There are problems with approaches that seek explanations for individual behaviour in terms of the function they perform for larger systems, but Parsons nevertheless offers some important insights. The suggestion that the response of societies to strains within the social system is to 'invent new categories of sickness' may seem far-fetched. After all, modern medicine justifies its status as grounded in an objective, scientific tradition, as in this statement by the British Medical Association (BMA):

> The work and approach of the medical profession are based on scientific method, defining 'science' in the strictest sense of the word, namely the systematic observation of natural phenomena for the purpose of discovering laws governing these phenomena ... As an integral part of the society in which we live, scientific methodology is generally held to be an acceptable basis on which to set reliable judgements, free from overriding social values and political bias.
>
> (British Medical Association 1986: 61)

Social definitions of illness

Can it truly be said that social values do not impinge in any way on medical judgements? Six years before this BMA report was published, Ian Kennedy (later to Chair the Bristol Inquiry and the Healthcare Commission) used the example of homosexuality to illustrate how moral judgements can be presented as clinical ones (Kennedy 1981).

Regarded in the nineteenth century as a sin, homosexuality instead came to be regarded as an illness:

homosexuals, formerly considered to be sinners, were labelled as ill – not bad, but mad. Commitments to mental institutions, hormonal treatments, and castrations were used to deal with unwanted sexual behaviour ... Treatments for homosexual men – such as aversion therapy – continued until, and beyond, 1973, when the American Psychiatric Association redesignated homosexuality as non-pathological.

(Hart and Wellings 2002: 897)

Although the particular focus changes, the boundaries of medicine in areas such as sexuality remain controversial. An example of this arose in 1995, as a consequence of a decision by North West Lancashire Health Authority not to offer surgery for 'sex changes'. Three years later, three transsexuals were successful in a claim to the High Court that the health authority had wrongly refused them gender reassignment surgery. The three, living as women, objected to the fact that the health authority introduced a 'blanket ban' on the operation, as a result of which they were in an 'acutely distressed mental and physical state'. Their barrister told the court that the health authority had decided they should receive counselling to reconcile them with their biological condition but this, he said, only added to their distress (*Guardian* 10.11.98).

In his ruling, the judge concluded that the health authority's decision to refuse the operation was 'unlawful and irrational'. The decision was taken, he added, without consideration of 'the proper treatment of a recognised illness' (*Guardian* 22.12.98).

The health authority was able to appeal against this ruling to the next judicial tier, the Appeal Court. They did so, but only to find that the ruling of the High Court was upheld and the health authority was judged to have acted unlawfully. According to a newspaper report of the Appeal Court hearing:

> The health authority had argued that it was entitled to take into account its own 'scarce resources' and refuse funding if it meant that serious illnesses, such as heart disease, cancer, kidney cases, and Aids, were not covered. Lord Justice Auld said the authority's policy was flawed. It did not treat transsexualism as an illness but 'as an attitude or state of mind which does not warrant medical treatment'. He added that the authority's attitude to transsexuals amounted to a blanket policy against funding treatment for the condition 'because it does not believe in such treatment'. Lord Justice Buxton said that the authority had not shown 'rational consideration' before deciding to 'give no funding at all to a procedure supported by respectable clinicians and psychiatrists, which is said to be necessary in certain cases to relieve extreme mental distress'.
>
> The authority's chief executive told the newspaper: 'This was never done just because of the cost of the treatment. We are saying, we have so much money and we have to ensure it is used as effectively as possible.'
>
> (*Guardian* 30.07.99)

An extreme example of the contested status of certain diagnosis gained media attention in 2000, as an item in the *Guardian* newspaper reported:

> A surgeon who amputated the healthy limbs from two psychologically disturbed men at their request said yesterday that he saw nothing wrong with his actions.
>
> Robert Smith cut off the lower limbs of two patients during private operations at Falkirk and District Infirmary. The two men were suffering from an extremely rare form of body dysmorphic disorder known as apotemnophilia. Those suffering from the disease have an obsessive belief that their body is 'incomplete' with four limbs and will only be complete after amputation.
>
> 'My fear is that someone will injure themselves or kill themselves', he said. 'I have very serious concerns that they will go to an unlicensed practitioner or take the law into their own hands and lie down on a railway line or take a shotgun.'
>
> Mr Smith's patients, who he said were severely disabled by their disorder, had rigorous psychological and psychiatric evaluations before their operations.
>
> (*Guardian* 01.02.2000)

Parsons' suggestion that societies may 'invent new categories of illness' does not imply these are constructed out of nothing, or are imaginary. Instead, categorization as sickness provides a socially legitimate and acceptable definition. This is sometimes referred to as being socially constructed, meaning that the categories being used should not be regarded as ones fixed by nature, and immutable, but rather represent ways that people find for explaining phenomena.

Without a clinical diagnosis sufferers can be left feeling that their condition lacks credibility and legitimacy. By granting legitimacy to the condition, medical diagnosis can to some degree move responsibility from the person to the body. However, some illnesses continue to be perceived as a failure of the person and diagnosis can bring with it negative consequences. This brings us to the concept of stigma.

Illness and stigma: Erving Goffman

> The Greeks originated the term *stigma* to refer to bodily signs, cut or burnt into the body, which were designed to expose the bearer as a slave, a criminal, or social outcast, someone 'ritually polluted' who was to be avoided, especially in public places. However, today the term is applied more widely to any condition, attribute, trait, or behaviour that symbolically marks the bearer off as 'culturally unacceptable' or 'inferior' and has as its subjective referent the notion of shame or disgrace.
>
> (Williams 1987: 136)

A sociologist who has given close attention to the concept of stigma is Erving Goffman, who describes it as, 'a special kind of relationship between attribute and stereotype' (Goffman 1968: 14). Certain attributes or characteristics can be stigmatizing because they are associated with stereotyped, and frequently negative, attitudes. In a discussion on the relationship between stigma and social identity, Goffman suggests three different types of stigma:

First there are abominations of the body – the various physical deformities. Next there are blemishes of individual character perceived as weak will, domineering or unnatural passions, treacherous and rigid beliefs, and dishonesty, these being inferred from a known record of, for example, mental disorder, imprisonment, addiction, alcoholism, homosexuality, unemployment, suicidal attempts, and radical political behaviour. Finally there are the tribal stigma of race, nation, and religion.

(Goffman 1968: 14)

To illuminate the concept, the following employs three examples related to illness, the first of a bodily deformity and the other two of 'blemishes of character'. At this stage, attention will not be given to what Goffman regards as a third source of stigma, although it forms an element in later discussion on inequalities of access to health care services.

Stigma and the body

The first example is drawn from a study of patients undergoing treatment for psoriasis, a skin disorder that may be small and localized but can result in extensive lesions, affecting much of the body. Jobling suggests:

Skin disorders generally offer one of the most striking examples of 'stigmatizing illness' ... There is evidence for example that the biblical condition commonly translated as 'leprosy' was not in fact the disease now known as Hansen's disease, but rather psoriasis. Skin disease has connotations of shame and guilt in many cultures, and has long attracted social condemnation.

(Jobling 1988: 226)

Although the research reported by Jobling was mainly concerned to explore patients' experiences of treatment, it also includes accounts of the illness. When asked to describe the worst thing about having psoriasis, many patients referred to the feelings that went with the physical condition. Examples included:

Revulsion against one's body and a feeling of never being really clean. (Man, 69 years, with psoriasis for 20 years)

One always feels unclean. In my young days I would never expose myself to view. (Woman, 53 years, with psoriasis for 30 years)

One feels unclean – with the constant shower of scales. (Woman, 44 years, psoriasis for 24 years)

I have always felt a sense of shame. I feel it most when I look at my body. I try to hide it even from my friends, especially from friends in fact. But the scales make it difficult. It is such a dirty disease. (Woman, 70 years, psoriasis for 12 years)

Jobling argues that: 'psoriasis is not only a physical "biological" disorder, it is (in common with other skin disorders) a social and cultural phenomenon of considerable complexity. It must be seen as such, and dealt with a such, if a better quality of life is to be achieved for those directly affected by it' (Jobling 1988: 242).

Stigma and sexuality

The role of stigma in causing biological disorders to become social and cultural phenomena, and hence experienced in particular ways, is strikingly demonstrated with the example of HIV/AIDS. This example also provides a powerful illustration of Goffman's second source of stigma, 'blemishes of individual character'. When HIV/AIDS first gained public attention, despite having similar routes of transmission as Hepatitis B, it was judged very differently. Whereas Hepatitis B was seen as contracted primarily through blood, and posing particular risks to health care workers, HIV/AIDS was closely associated with sexuality. Although some other groups were identified as having high rates of the disease, including Haitians and injecting drug users, it was predominantly constructed and perceived as a sexual disease.

The significance of this was reflected in early newspaper reports of cases of infection through contaminated blood used in transfusions. One British newspaper ran a story on this under the headline:

> AIDS: Why Should the Innocent Suffer?
>
> (*Daily Express* 25.09.85)

The implication is that those who contracted the disease through sexual contact were in some way 'guilty'. The distinction between 'guilty' and 'innocent' victims is an enormously important one, introducing a profoundly moral dimension to the perception of illness. This moral dimension was reflected in jokes circulating among gay men in the United States in the early 1980s, expressing the stigma associated with the disease with wry humour:

> Hi mom, I've got bad news and good. The bad news is, I'm gay. The good news is, I'm dying.
>
> What's the hardest thing about having AIDS? Trying to convince your mother that you're Haitian.
>
> (Quoted in Goldstein 1991: 26)

In a discussion on early cultural responses to HIV/AIDS, Richard Goldstein, the arts editor of the New York alternative magazine, *Village Voice*, stresses the role of the anxieties it aroused:

> AIDS arrived in the midst of a moral (and political) panic over sexuality. The assumption that medicine had conquered venereal disease was replaced by an ominous revelation: science could not contain a new and deadly sexually transmitted disease. If anything, technological sophistication added to the

anxiety by making AIDS seem unlike any previous pandemic. Here was an illness whose long latency differentiated it from influenza or plague, which could sweep through a population in only weeks. Now, it was possible to ascertain that infection occurred years before the onset of disease. This 'diagnosis' created a new class of 'patients', forced to live between sickness and health, giving a tangible twist to the old medical term, 'worried well'.

(Goldstein 1991: 38–9)

It is difficult to comprehend the enormous amount of moral energy some people expend in coping with other people's sexuality, especially when this indignation could be directed so easily towards problems of poverty, malnutrition and injustice. However it is explained, it illustrates the scope for moral judgements to be applied to illness.

Stigma and mental health

Mental illness, particularly when generating behaviours which may seem unpredictable and inexplicable, can also be a source of stigma. The British government has recently announced plans to challenge the stigma and discrimination that people with mental illness can face, an intention broadly welcomed by organizations working in this area. Angela Greatley, acting chief executive of the Sainsbury Centre for Mental Health at the time of writing, has responded:

Having a mental health problem does not in itself prevent a person from having a home, a job or an education. It is only because people with mental health problems are sidelined by others in our society that they so often face a downward spiral of ill health, poverty and isolation. This spiral must be broken as a matter of urgency.

(BBC News, 13 June 2004)

However, Dr Mike Shooter, President of the Royal College of Psychiatrists has expressed concern that other aspects of government policy may reinforce the stigma associated with mental illness. His comments relate to the proposal to allow individuals with 'personality disorders' to be detained, even if no treatment is available and they have committed no crime:

We are concerned that the proposed new Mental Health Bill will actually increase the stigma associated with mental illness, by focusing on risk. It is vital that this report has a positive impact on the lives of people with mental health problems both in terms of improving the legislation and tackling discrimination.

('Bid to end mental health stigma', BBC News, 13 June 2004)

At a time when it has become fashionable in some quarters to denounce what is pejoratively referred to as 'political correctness', it is worth noting the continuing potential for language to stigmatize. An example comes from a publication produced by the Electoral Commission, the body responsible for overseeing electoral arrangements in the UK. The issue concerned the means by which people are judged capable of voting, in the context of mental illness and learning disabilities. In advice to electoral administrators, the Commission used language which has long passed out of everyday speech but still retains a meaning in law. Specifically, it pointed out that among those who are not allowed to vote in the UK are: 'people with mental disabilities if, on polling day, they are incapable of making a reasoned judgement ("idiots" and "lunatics")'.

The guidelines stated that the eligibility of someone with a profound disability could be questioned: 'because under the common law so-called "idiots" cannot vote ... So-called "lunatics" on the other hand can vote, though only in their lucid intervals, and so could not be excluded from the register on this ground.'

Attention was drawn to the issue when a member of the Northern Ireland Assembly, Patsy McGlone of the Social Democratic Labour Party, tried to get a constituent with Down syndrome onto the electoral register: 'It's incredible that something so insulting to these people and their families should appear' he said (*Financial Times* 14.04.04).

Whether or not the application of a diagnostic label leads to stigma, it does mark someone as different. As we saw, it was Parsons' view that medical diagnosis represents a socially functional means of dealing with deviance, but why should medical labels, rather than those of some other form, play this role? This is a question addressed by writers who believe too much of everyday life has been appropriated by medicine.

Illness and 'medicalization': Irving Zola and Ivan Illich

In the early 1970s, an American sociologist, Irving Zola, argued that medicine was becoming: 'the new repository of truth, the place where absolute and often final judgements are made by supposedly morally neutral and objective experts' (Zola 1972 in Cox and Mead 1975: 170). In doing so, he suggests, it is: 'nudging aside, if not incorporating, the more traditional institutions of religion and law' (Zola 1972 in Cox and Mead 1975: 170).

This, he argued, is being achieved by a process of 'medicalizing' much of everyday living. He presents this not as a 'definite argument' but a 'case in progress', but he believed too many normal human experiences were being classified as illness. A consequence of this was that medicine was increasingly assuming responsibility for areas of life in which it was inappropriate:

> By the very acceptance of a specific behaviour as an 'illness' and the definition of illness as an undesirable state, the issue becomes not whether to deal with a particular problem, but *how* and *when*. Thus the debate over homosexuality, drugs or abortion becomes focused on the degree of sickness attached to the phenomenon in question or the extent of the health risk involved. And the more principled, more perplexing, or even moral issue of what freedom an individual should have over his or her own body is shunted aside.
>
> (Zola 1972, in Cox and Mead 1975: 182)

The medicalizing of society

Zola describes this process as the 'medicalizing of society':

> From sex to food, from aspirins to clothes, from driving your car to riding the surf, it seems that under certain conditions, or in combination with certain other substances or activities or if done too much or too little, virtually anything can lead to certain medical problems. In short, I at least have finally been convinced that living is injurious to health. This remark is not meant as facetiously as it may sound. But rather every aspect of our daily life has in it elements of risk to health.
>
> These facts take on particular importance not only when health becomes a paramount value in society, but also a phenomenon whose diagnosis and treatment has been restricted to a certain group. For this means that that group, perhaps unwittingly, is in a position to exercise great control and influence about what we should and should not do to attain that 'paramount value'.
>
> (Zola 1972, in Cox and Mead 1975: 180)

The last paragraph reflects two of Zola's fundamental concerns. The first is that 'health' has become disproportionately important in relation to other aims and values. He is not suggesting health is unimportant but that it is not simply an end in itself:

> Nor does it really matter if we were guaranteed six more inches in height, thirty more years of life or drugs to expand our potentialities and potencies; we should still be able to ask, what do six inches matter, in what kind of environment will the thirty additional years be spent, or who will decide what potentialities and potencies will be expanded and what curbed
>
> (Zola 1972, in Cox and Mead 1975: 184)

Zola's second concern is that these issues come to be seen as the responsibility of the medical profession. His claim was not so much that this is the outcome of a desire by the medical profession to strengthen its influence, but that people's own anxieties are moving things in this direction: 'the most powerful empirical stimulus for this is the realization of how much everyone has or believes he has something organically wrong with him, or put more positively, how much can be done to make one feel, look or function better' (Zola 1972, in Cox and Mead 1975: 179).

Zola feared that it would always be possible to find evidence of ill-health if one looked hard enough. There is a considerable amount of evidence that supports this proposition. One early example, referred to by Scheff (1963), looked at decisions by doctors in the 1940s about performing tonsillectomies on children. The study was based on a group of 1000 children and:

> Of these, some 611 had had their tonsils removed. The remaining 389 were then examined by other physicians, and 174 were selected for tonsillectomy.

This left 215 children whose tonsils were apparently normal. Another group of doctors was put to work examining these 215 children, and 99 of them were adjudged in need of tonsillectomy. Still another group of doctors was then employed to examine the remaining children, and nearly one-half were recommended for operation.

(Scheff 1963, in Tuckett and Kaufert 1978: 249)

The potential for people's anxieties to interact with the ability of clinical diagnosis to identify a 'problem' led Zola to conclude that modern medicine was extending its reach too far. This, he felt, assumes particular importance:

not only when health becomes a paramount value in society, but also a phenomenon whose diagnosis and treatment has been restricted to a certain group. For this means that that group, perhaps unwittingly, is in a position to exercise great control and influence about what we should and should not do to attain that 'paramount value'.

(Zola 1972, in Cox and Mead 1975: 180)

Ivan Illich and 'Medical Nemesis'

Nemesis, in Greek mythology the goddess of retribution and vengeance, provides Ivan Illich with a symbol for what he saw as the damage done by medicine. Illich was not a sociologist but launched a trenchant critique of Western medicine that provides some valuable challenges. Born in Vienna in 1926, Ivan Illich studied theology and philosophy at the Gregorian University in Rome before obtaining a PhD in history. Moving to the United States he became an assistant-pastor in an Irish-Puerto Rican parish in New York, before becoming vice-rector to the Catholic University of Puerto Rico in 1956, a position he held until 1960.

In 1976 his book, *Limits to Medicine: Medical Nemesis*, was published in Britain, in which a footnote indicates that he became aware of Zola's article on medicalization only after reading the final proofs of his own book: 'and I was unable to indicate that the term "medicalization" of society in the sense in which I use it in this book had been applied to the same phenomenon in this brilliant and dense essay' (Illich 1976: 48).

Iatrogenic illness

A starting point for appreciating the argument advanced by Illich is the notion of iatrogenic illness. This is used to describe illness that is caused by medicine itself, and forms a central theme of Illich's book. Illich begins his account by considering clinical iatrogenesis. This occurs where a treatment has undesirable side effects, or unintended consequences, as in hospital-acquired infection. This use of the idea of iatrogenic illness is important, but not particularly novel: Illich's more radical thinking is evident in the ways he extends the concept to embrace other forms.

Social iatrogenesis

One other form is the notion of social iatrogenesis, which he asserts exists:

> when health care is turned into a standardized item, a staple; when all suffering is 'hospitalized' and homes become inhospitable to birth, sickness, and death; when the language in which people could experience their bodies is turned into bureaucratic gobbledegook; or when suffering, mourning and healing outside the patient role are labelled a form of deviance.
>
> (Illich 1976: 49)

Part of Illich's case is built on the burgeoning cost of health care, particularly that which is delivered through hospitals, although he notes the tighter constraints on spending that applied in the British National Health Service compared to the system in the United States. Only in China, he argues, does the trend at first sight seem to run in the opposite direction, with an emphasis upon primary care provided by non-professional technicians. However, he warns, investment is being directed increasingly towards a 'well qualified and highly orthodox medical profession': 'barefoot medicine', he suggests, 'is losing its makeshift, semi-independent, grassroots character and is being integrated into a unitary health-care technocracy' (Illich 1976: 67).

Although he discusses the role of professional monopolies, Illich is more interested in people's demand for health care:

> More and more people subconsciously know that they are sick and tired of their jobs and of their leisure passivities, but they want to hear the lie that physical illness relieves them of social and political responsibilities. They want their doctor to act as lawyer and priest. As a lawyer, the doctor exempts the patient from his normal duties and enables him to cash in on the insurance fund he was forced to build. As a priest, he becomes the patient's accomplice in creating the myth that he is an innocent victim of biological mechanisms rather than a lazy, greedy, or envious deserter of a social struggle for control over the tools of production. Social life becomes a giving and receiving of therapy: medical, psychiatric, pedagogic, or geriatric. Claiming access to treatment becomes a political duty, and medical certification a powerful device for social control.
>
> (Illich 1976: 129–30)

Cultural iatrogenesis

Turning to Illich's third form of iatrogenesis, we come to what he sees emerging when 'the medical enterprise saps the will of people to suffer their reality' (Illich 1976: 133). Cultural iatrogenesis is regarded by Illich as a manifestation of modern society whereby pain and suffering are seen as problems to be managed or produced out of existence, rather than 'an inevitable part of their conscious coping with reality' (p. 140). A consequence of this, he asserts, is that: 'The so-called health professions have an even deeper, culturally health-denying effect in so far as they destroy the potential of people to deal with their human weakness, vulnerability, and uniqueness in a personal and autonomous way' (Illich 1976: 42).

Illich deals with three areas where he believes cultural iatrogenesis is evident: the 'killing of pain', the 'invention and elimination of disease' and the experience of death. His view can be illustrated with some brief comments on the first two of these.

Culture and pain

On the tendency to seek ways of avoiding pain, Illich uses the example of childbirth to point to the important role that culture can play in pain: 'culture decrees whether the mother or father or both must groan when the child is born' (Illich 1976: 143).

Illich's thinking on this issue had been influenced by the work of Grantly Dick-Read, particularly his book 1942 book, *Childbirth Without Fear*. Developing his views from working in a private gynaecology practice in London, Dick-Read was strongly critical of moves towards the almost routine use of anaesthetic during labour. While not rejecting pain relief, he believed there was an association between fear, muscular tension and the pain that was experienced. Rather than use anaesthetics as standard, Dick-Read advocated the use of psychological and physical exercises, focusing on breathing, relaxation and self-assurance. Despite 'provoking anger from much of the medical establishment' (Porter 1997: 696), Dick-Read's 1942 book became a best-seller, and was translated into ten languages. In Britain, many of his ideas were taken up by the National Childbirth Trust, established in 1956, and: 'in the Soviet Union "psychoprophylaxis" – learning to ignore pain by concentrating on somatic sensations elsewhere – was adopted in 1951 as the official method of childbirth pain relief' (Porter 1997: 697).

The 'invention of disease'

A second area where Illich believed cultural iatrogenesis had an impact was in 'the invention and elimination of disease'. Noting the work on mental illness of diverse writers such as Erving Goffman, Thomas Szasz and R.D. Laing, Illich criticizes a tendency to question the existential status of mental illness by contrasting it with 'real' physical illness. Challenging this, he argues that categories of physical disease are no more 'real', developing this to maintain that clinical diagnosis diverts attention from the real source of tension:

> As long as disease is something that takes possession of people, something they 'catch' or 'get', the victims of these natural processes can be exempted from responsibility for their condition ... An advanced industrial society is sick-making because it disables people from coping with their environment and, when they break down, it substitutes a 'clinical' prosthesis for the broken *relationships*. People would rebel against such an environment if medicine did not explain their biological disorientation as a defect in their health, rather than

as a defect in the way of life which is imposed on them or which they impose on themselves.

(Illich 1976: 173–4)

The concept of medicalization is an important one, although there are considerable differences in the way in which the term is used by Zola and Illich, on the one hand, and Cornwell on the other. Both Zola and Illich are concerned that people are abandoning their own responsibilities by passing to doctors the right to decide on their condition and behaviour. It is not necessary to take such a negative view of medicine – Cornwell, for instance, does not share it – to acknowledge that medicine does play an increasingly important part in explaining the human condition. However, since the early 1970s there have been substantial challenges to medical authority, and medical expertise is no longer automatically accepted on trust.

The situation today may be considerably different from the time when the 'medicalization thesis' was first proposed. Although not particularly emphasizing the notion of 'consumer', Zola and Illich were interested in the role patients, and potential patients, were playing in extending the boundaries of medicine. Increasingly today we may need to supplement this focus upon the relationship between the patient and the professional to also take account of commercial interests.

From medicalization to commercialization?

Critics of modern medicine, such as Ivan Illich and Irving Zola, were writing on the eve of a period that witnessed what the historian Harold Perkin describes as a 'backlash against professional society' (Perkin 1989). Much of the twentieth century saw the authority of many professional groups increasing, but by its closing years this tide had begun to ebb. The 1980s and 1990s saw a host of government policies designed to constrain and manage professional autonomy, and as we enter the twenty-first century, it is commercial interests that may require much greater scrutiny and critique.

Writing in 1980, the editor of the *New England Journal of Medicine*, Arnold Relman, referred to the 'new medical industrial complex' as: 'the most important recent development in American health care' (cited in Salmon 1984: 144).

Echoing the notion of corporate America as a 'military industrial complex', what he had in mind was a process in which:

nationwide and multinational corporations will become prominent providers of healthcare services, with their primary purpose being profit. The rapidity and scope of this trend in the organization of health care is phenomenal in that proprietary corporate forms only began in the US in the late 1960s.

(Salmon 1984: 143)

The control of health care provision by large private companies in the United States is very different to the situation in the UK, where the National Health

Service remains the main provider. However, the present New Labour Government is encouraging the boundaries between the NHS and private providers to become blurred, and several commentators are noting the greater role this is giving the private sector (see, for example, Pollock, 2004).

Organizational developments of this type are not the only means by which commercial interests are gaining prominence. More fundamental is their role in developing treatments for illnesses, and even stimulating the construction of new categories of illness. In this, the pharmaceutical industry deserves particular attention.

Two decades ago, an American physician and academic, Thomas Bodenheimer claimed: 'The expansion of profit-motivated capitalist enterprise into the pharmaceutical area has turned its life-giving potential into at best a mixed, at worst a negative factor for the people of the world' (Bodenheimer 1984: 203).

There are several strands to this assertion and attention here is restricted to the argument that pharmaceutical companies become inappropriately involved in developing and defining new categories of illness. This is a claim made by an Australian journalist, Ray Moynihan, who argues:

> There's a lot of money to be made from telling healthy people they're sick. Some forms of medicalising ordinary life may now be better described as disease mongering: widening the boundaries of treatable illness in order to expand markets for those who sell and deliver treatments. Pharmaceutical companies are actively involved in sponsoring the definition of diseases and promoting them to both prescribers and consumers. The social construction of illness is being replaced by the corporate construction of disease.
>
> (Moynihan, Heath and Henry 2002: 886)

The claim can be illustrated by referring to three examples, female sexual dysfunction, irritable bowel disease and social phobia.

Female sexual dysfunction

Moynihan refers to an article, published in February 1999 in the *Journal of the American Medical Association* entitled, 'Sexual dysfunction in the United States: prevalence and predictors' (Moynihan 2003). This reported that 43 per cent of women aged 18–59 experienced sexual dysfunction, a figure subsequently repeated in other material. Moynihan is concerned that two of the report authors had connections with the pharmaceutical company Pfizer, which was seeking to develop a female equivalent to its drug used to treat erection difficulties, sildenafil (Viagra).

Moynihan argues there are serious doubts about the accuracy of the figure quoted, essentially arising from the way 'dysfunction' is defined. In the study from which the figure was drawn, in which 1500 women were asked about sexual experiences in the preceding 12 months, all who answered positively to any one of seven questions were included. Among these were women who described occasions when they had felt a lack of desire for sex, had anxieties about their own sexual performance, or had experienced difficulties with lubrication. Should these really be described as 'dysfunctional'?

An important contributor to research in this area, Dr Irwin Goldstein, nevertheless regularly cites the 43 per cent prevalence figure as justification for developing models of 'vaginal engorgement insufficiency and clitoral erectile insufficiency'. The basis of these findings, according to Moynihan, has been provided by studies of female New Zealand white rabbits!

Emotional or psychological experiences will often be accompanied by physiological changes but cannot be reduced to them. How are experiences such as a lack of desire for sex, anxiety about sexual performance and difficulties with lubrication to be understood and explained? Moynihan notes that Dr John Bancroft, the director of the Kinsey Institute at Indiana University, regards the term 'dysfunction' in this context as highly misleading:

> The danger of portraying sexual difficulties as a dysfunction is that it is likely to encourage doctors to prescribe drugs to change sexual function – when the attention should be paid to other aspects of the woman's life. It's also likely to make women think they have a malfunction when they do not.
>
> (Moynihan 2003: 46)

Moynihan concludes: 'These revelations about female sexual dysfunction should spark a more widespread and rigorous investigation into the role of drug companies in defining and promoting new diseases and disorders' (Moynihan 2003: 47).

Irritable bowel syndrome

A second example, drawn from Australia, is the condition of irritable bowel syndrome (Moynihan, Heath and Henry 2002). A leaked document, produced by a communications company on behalf of GlaxoSmithKline (the manufacturers of the drug Lotronex (alosetron hydrochloride)) describes the planning of a 'medical education' programme with clearly specified objectives: 'IBS (Irritable Bowel Syndrome) must be established in the minds of doctors as a significant and discrete disease state' (Moynihan, Heath and Henry 2002).

Other groups to be targeted with promotional material include pharmacists, nurses and patients. The latter, it suggests, 'need to be convinced that IBS is a common and recognised medical disorder'. A 'patient support programme' is also proposed, to enable GlaxoSmithKline to, 'reap the loyalty dividend when the competitor drug kicks in' (Moynihan, Heath and Henry 2002).

Detailed description of the programme includes proposals to establish an Advisory Board, comprising 'key opinion leaders' from across Australia, to advise the company on current opinions in gastroenterology and 'opportunities for shaping it'. It was important to have this credibility, it is suggested, so that GPs are reassured 'that the material they receive is clinically valid'. The whole thrust of the programme is oriented towards what is described as establishing the condition as a 'serious and credible disease'.

Owing to developments elsewhere, with the United States Food and Drugs Administration reporting serious and sometimes fatal adverse reactions to Lotronex, the drug was withdrawn. Nevertheless, Moynihan *et al.* argue that the example illustrates how: 'staff and organisations sponsored by a drug company are helping to shape medical and public opinion about the condition the company is targeting with its new product' ((Moynihan, Heath and Henry 2002).

Social phobia

The third example concerns the marketing strategies adopted to support the antidepressant Aurorix (moclobemide) produced by Roche and, in particular, the promotion of 'social phobia' as a clinical condition susceptible to treatment by the drug. This strategy is described in a guide published by the British magazine, *Pharmaceutical Marketing*:

> You may even need to reinforce the actual existence of a disease and/or the value of treating it. A classic example of this was the need to create recognition in Europe of social phobia as a distinct clinical entity and the potential of antidepressant agents such as moclobemide to treat it.

It adds: 'Social phobia was recognised in the US and so transatlantic opinion leaders were mobilised to participate in advisory activities, meetings, publications etc. to help influence the overall belief in Europe' (quoted in Moynihan, Heath and Henry 2002).

Social phobia was first described as a diagnostic classification in 1980 and now represents the third most common psychiatric disorder in the United States (after major depression and alcohol dependence). However, D. Double, a consultant psychiatrist, claims that 'social phobia' or 'social anxiety disorder' 'could be seen as the process of medicalizing shyness'. Noting that the number of diagnostic categories in the *Diagnostic and Statistical Manual of Mental Disorders of the American Psychiatric Association* rose from 106 in 1952 to 357 in 1994, Double suggests: 'We should be sceptical about the potency and benefits of drugs for this condition' (Double 2002: 902).

Advertising prescription drugs direct to the public

In response to their critics, pharmaceutical companies have mounted a robust defence. A joint article by a Vice-President and Executive Director of the drug manufacturer Merck claims that diseases are in fact both underdiagnosed and undertreated. To help overcome this, they urge allowing direct advertising of prescription-only medicines to the public, rather than restricting this to professional journals. In Europe the pharmaceutical industry is not able to communicate directly with consumers in this way:

> whereas other people are free to disseminate information of perhaps dubious quality. European citizens deserve access to balanced, accurate, evidence

based, and comprehensive information about the healthcare choices they face
– when and how they wish.

(Bonaccorso and Sturchio 2002: 910)

Bonaccorso and Sturchio argue that doctors today are dealing with more
informed patients, who are taking greater responsibility for making choices in
consultation with their doctors. Increasing the amount of advertising for prescription-only items that is directed to the consumer, they claim: 'may well shift the
balance of control in the consultation ... The quality of the consultation can only
be enhanced by the widening and deepening of the patient's knowledge in this
way' (Bonaccorso and Sturchio 2002: 910).

The objection that the companies will offer biased information, because their
desire will be to increase their market share, meets the response that other sources
may also be biased – with professionals seeking to protect their authority and
territory, and governments wanting to control budgets, for example. It is con-
descending they suggest, to assume that consumers will not recognize the different
agendas held by each group (Bonaccorso and Sturchio 2002).

Others argue that public advertising of this form leads to inappropriate
treatment. Mintzes refers to a report by the Dutch Health Inspectorate showing
dramatic increases in consultations for toenail fungus after a three-month media
campaign. Similarly, during a campaign for the hair stimulating drug finasteride
(Propecia) in the US in 1998, visits to doctors for baldness rose by 79 per cent
above levels of the previous year (Mintzes 2002).

Moynihan, Heath and Henry (2002) report a double-page advertisement,
published in Australia, which claimed 39 per cent of men who visited their GP had
erection problems. The advertisement did not explain that the figure came from a
study that included all who reported any problems, even if only 'occasionally'. The
average age of those reporting complete erectile dysfunction was 71. The advertisement carried the name of an organization concerned about the condition,
Impotence Australia, but did not mention it was established with funding from the
pharmaceutical company Pfizer. In correspondence with the authors of the article,
a spokesperson for Pfizer defended the company's actions by arguing: 'The best
consumer is an educated consumer ... Who better than the manufacturer to help
this process?' (Quoted in Moynihan, Health and Henry 2002: 889).

Choice, power and knowledge

Whether or not this claim is one that British Government ministers at the time of
writing would want to endorse, the underlying argument resonates with their own
emphasis upon expanding patient choice and treating the patient as a customer.
Indeed, from this perspective the arguments of the manufacturers may appear
reasonable. Preventing the public from seeing such advertisements can be seen as
an extreme form of paternalism. How can it be right to prevent people having
access to information that assists the making of informed choices?

This example illustrates why we should think clearly about notions such as
paternalism and choice. The possession of technical knowledge can provide a

significant source of social power; and how it is communicated and shared with others is an important building block in constructing relationships with those to whom it is applied. This raises quite fundamental questions about how information should be handled, and who should be responsible for its dissemination. In relation to pharmaceutical products, this has especial salience given the scale of current spending. In the UK, and other OECD countries, the percentage of public spending on pharmaceuticals as a percentage of Gross Domestic Product rose from 0.4 per cent in 1970 to 0.7 per cent in 1996. In same period, the proportion of NHS spending on pharmaceuticals rose from 12.5 per cent to 16.1 per cent (Freemantle and Hill 2002).

It is worth noting that Ivan Illich considers but rejects the argument that the pharmaceutical companies are to blame for 'medicalization'. Maintaining that it is the medical profession, not the search for corporate profits, that is responsible, he comments:

> the per capita use of medically prescribed drugs around the world seems to have little to do with commercial promotion; it correlates mostly with the number of doctors, even in socialist countries where the education of physicians is not influenced by drug industry publicity and where corporate drug-pushing is limited.
>
> (Illich 1976: 81)

Despite his rejection of the argument that commercial rather than professional interests are dominant, Illich makes some chilling observations on a political experiment in Chile in the early 1970s:

> One doctor in Latin America who was also a statesman did try to stem the pharmaceutical invasion rather than just enlist physicians to make it look respectable. During his short tenure as president of Chile, Dr Salvador Allende quite successfully mobilized the poor to identify their own health needs and much less successfully compelled the medical profession to serve basic rather than profitable needs. He proposed to ban drugs unless they had been tried on paying clients in North America or Europe for as long as the patent protection would run. He revived a programme aimed at reducing the national pharmacopoeia to a few dozen items, more or less the same as those carried by the Chinese barefoot doctor in his black wicker box. Notably, within one week after the Chilean military junta took power on 11 September 1973, many of the most outspoken proponents of Chilean medicine based on community action rather than on drug imports and drug consumption had been murdered.
>
> (Illich 1976: 77)

Commercial interests provide yet another route by which personal troubles and public issues become connected. Pharmaceutical and biotechnology companies are gaining immense economic and political power. Without neglecting the continuing role and influence of professional authority, the increasing ability of commercial interests to shape the environment in which these operate needs to be acknowledged.

The four examples considered here – illness as deviance, medicalization, stigma and the commercialization of illness – all represent ways of understanding the relationship between the personal and the social, the private and the public. They are not alternatives but offer different and possibly complementary perspectives. They can help us understand the context in which patients and professionals meet; the focus for the next chapter.

5
Patients, clients and professionals

This chapter draws together themes from earlier ones, particularly the role of different kinds of knowledge, and applies these to the interaction that occurs between the patient and professional. While these encounters provide the main focus for the chapter, it is important to acknowledge, as Margaret Stacey has pointed out in relation to medicine, that the idea of one-to-one relationships between patients and professionals is rarely accurate (Stacey 1992). In reality, professionals typically work as part of a larger team.

The historian, Harold Perkin, describes the traditional client–professional relationship as characterized by the 'condescension of professionalism'. By this he means:

> The professional *had* to assert the high quality and scarcity value of the service he provided or forgo the status and rewards that went with it. And since that service took a personal form it could not be detached from the superior person who provided it. This indeed was the Achilles' heel of professionalism, through which entered the spears of individual arrogance, collective condescension towards the laity, and mutual disdain between the different professions.
>
> (Perkin 1989: 390)

There may be some accuracy in this statement but there is another important dimension to acknowledge. This is summed up in the notion of 'paternalism' and is epitomized in the model of the 'sick role' proposed by Talcott Parsons in the 1950s.

The 'sick role' and the legacy of paternalism

As has previously been described, Parsons' starting point was the concept of a social system and the mechanisms by which it maintains equilibrium. In modern society, he saw sickness as an increasingly important response to people's problems with coping, and that a crucial role is played by the medical profession in classifying it as legitimate. It is the meeting of the patient with the doctor that presents Parsons with an opportunity to develop what he refers to as the 'sick role'.

His conception of this puts considerable emphasis on the dependency of the patient:

> By institutional definition of the sick role the sick person is helpless and therefore in need of help. If being sick is to be regarded as 'deviant' as certainly in important respects it must, it is ... distinguished from other deviant roles precisely by the fact that the sick person is not regarded as 'responsible' for his condition, 'he can't help it'. He may, of course, have carelessly exposed himself to danger of accident, but then once injured he cannot, for instance, mend a fractured leg by 'will power' ...
>
> By the same institutional definition the sick person is not, of course, competent to help himself, or what he can do is, except for trivial illness, not adequate. But in our culture there is a special definition of the kind of help he needs, namely, professional, technically competent help. The nature of this help imposes a further disability or handicap upon him. He is not only generally not in a position to do what needs to be done, but he does not 'know' what needs to be done or how to do it ...
>
> Only a technically trained person has that qualification. And one of the most serious disabilities of the layman is that he is not qualified to judge technical qualifications, in general or in detail. Two physicians may very well give conflicting diagnoses of the same case, indeed often do. In general the layman is not qualified to choose between them. Nor is he qualified to choose the 'best' physician among a panel. If he were fully rational he would have to rely on professional authority, on the advice of the professionally qualified or on institutional validation.
>
> Finally, third, the situation of illness very generally presents the patient and those close to him with complex problems of emotional adjustment.
>
> (Parsons, quoted in Bocock and Thompson 1992: 202–3)

Professional control

The dependency that Parsons saw as inherent in the professional–patient relationship was interpreted by another sociologist, Eliot Freidson, as the basis for professional control. Freidson did not share the emphasis upon the functional benefits suggested by Parsons, and instead suggests that in the kind of model that was dominant patients are likely to:

> develop new organization of their lives, an organization flowing from the professionally-defined demands of their treatment ... develop a round of life tempered by their own view of their illness and organized by the demands of regular professional observation and treatment of their difficulty. It is important to bear in mind that such a round of life is *not* organized by the disease and the biological incapacity it may produce, but by the professional

conceptions of the disease and what is needed to treat it: the disease becomes a professionally organized illness.

(Freidson 1975: 311–12)

Freidson pays particular attention to experiences of chronic illness and is critical of a professional style now often described as paternalistic. The concept of paternalism features in two major inquiries into care within the NHS, one relating to paediatric cardiac services at Bristol and the other to the removal and storage of body organs at Alder Hey Hospital, Liverpool. Neither inquiry was concerned about providing a sociological analysis but both came to conclusions that are important for understanding the sociology of patient–practitioner relationships.

A paternalistic style, limiting the scope for individual choice in the supposed best interest of the person to whom it is being applied, is evident in the following advice issued for pregnant women by the British Medical Association in the 1970s:

You decide when to see your doctor and let him confirm the fact of your pregnancy. From then onwards you are going to have to answer a lot of questions and be the subject of a lot of examinations. Never worry about any of these. They are necessary, they are in the interests of your baby and yourself, and none of them will ever hurt you.

(BMA 1977, cited in Open University 1985: 62)

Patient access to medical records

The phrase 'be the subject of' conveys a sense of passivity and dependency. Similar attitudes were revealed in a study exploring consultants' attitudes towards patients having access to their own general practice records (Britten 1991). The study included interviews with 24 consultants; 11 opposed the policy, with ten in favour and three ambivalent about it. With such a small sample the numbers themselves are unimportant, but the results indicated that the major factor determining these consultants' views was how they perceived the competence of patients in taking an active and informed role:

The views of the consultants opposed to access were that patients are not competent. By portraying patients in derogatory terms and by describing those who wanted access as difficult, they presented the patient as disqualified from full participation in the consultation.

(Britten 1991: 87)

Examples of this type of view included the following:

If we feel a patient is lying or is lazy or malingering on one side of things or if we feel they've got a very bad outlook and our treatment is a waste of time or they're not going to be compliant or there are social problems, all those things are going to have to be skirted around.

... the neurotic, stupid, irritating patients ... the patients who habitually complain, habitually preoccupied with their own health, often with minor things ...

The sort of person who wants to see their notes has got problems anyway.

The patients who take up a lot of time with questions that are off the point rather than to the point I'm sure would be the people who would be rifling through their notes at the first opportunity.

Consultants opposed to patients having access to their own records were also likely to believe that they were better placed than patients to make decisions. Typically, this would be presented as being in the best interests of the patient:

I think we're entitled to present such information as we've got for the patient's benefit. For example, if we've got a patient whom we know is going to die within three months but is perfectly well at the moment, to go and say 'go off and write your will, you've only got three months left' ... I think is not good.

I think somebody wouldn't want to know they'd been tested for syphilis if they hadn't got it.

Associated with this was a view that patients simply did not need to know all the information possessed by the doctor:

So I think it isn't necessary for patients to understand how or why they've been treated in a particular way or what diagnosis or formulation the doctor has made, it isn't necessary for patients to have total direct unlimited access to their notes.

Two other factors distinguishing doctors who were for and against access were attitudes towards whether patients should always be told the truth, and towards the fallibility of medicine (Britten 1991). These are matters on which current guidance from professional bodies has changed substantially since the 1960s and 1970s. Compare, for instance, the advice from the BMA to pregnant women given in 1977 with the following guidance to doctors on how to go about obtaining consent from patients for surgical and other interventions, given by the General Medical Council in 1998: 'It is for the patient, not the doctor, to determine what is in the patient's own best interests ... you may wish to recommend a treatment or a course of action, but you must not put pressure on patients to accept your advice.'

Paternalism and trust

That said, debates continue as to whether this represents the right approach. T.B. Brewin, a retired consultant oncologist, has put the case for retaining a measure of paternalism, emphasizing the importance of trust:

We need to strike a balance between 'informed consent' and 'paternalism'. The idea of the first as a great good and the second as a great evil is today in danger of being carried to absurd lengths. Yet few doctors dare say so (at any rate in public) for fear of being called paternalistic, old-fashioned, arrogant – or worse.

(Brewin 1995)

Brewin takes issue with those who argue that for consent to be meaningful it must be based upon the receipt of full information. He claims this neglects the role that trust plays in any relationship between experts and those they serve. This is linked with a view that explaining an unnecessary amount of detail to every patient wastes time that could be spent on patient care in far more valuable ways. Brewin also notes the variability between patients in the amount of information they require, objecting that 'anti-paternalists' seem to believe that every patient should be treated alike, with no account taken of the fact that what is right for one person may not be so for another:

What we need is better communication; more explanation for those who need it, less for those who don't; and greater empathy and understanding of the patient's real needs, fears, and aspirations. What we don't need is unhelpful rhetoric; a wholesale attack on trust; excessive emphasis on 'fully informed consent' and 'autonomy'; and a serious distortion of priorities with a consequent fall in standards of care.

For two reasons there has to be a compromise. Firstly, because noble principles often give contradictory advice. Every patient has a right to full information. He also has a right to be treated with compassion, common sense, and respect for his dignity – a respect that is not usually enhanced by asking him, 'Do you want us to be frank about all the risks or not?' Secondly, because we are all prisoners of time, the more time we spend trying to explain things, the less there is for other aspects of patient care.

Who should make the compromise? Presumably it should be those members of society who have most experience of all the subtle and paradoxical ways in which human beings may react to illness and to fear; and who have had the greatest opportunity of learning, from first hand experience, when to speak out and when to keep silent. In other words, doctors and nurses, rather than philosophers or experts in ethics.

(Brewin 1995: 355–6)

Although, as Brewin's remarks indicate, conventional thinking on these matters has changed, this does not necessarily mean there has been an equal shift in behaviour. Relatively recent inquiries into serious incidents at the Royal Bristol Infirmary and at Alder Hey Hospital found evidence of paternalistic styles, with the Bristol inquiry demonstrating that this could have consequences for clinical outcomes.

Paediatric Cardiac Services Inquiry

The inquiry into Paediatric Cardiac Services (PCS) in Bristol was prompted by concerns that clinical outcomes were inferior to comparable services elsewhere in the country. The report noted that in many ways the service provided at Bristol was 'adequate or more than adequate' and that the great majority of children who underwent surgery are alive. The dedication and commitment of staff is also recognized, as is the fact that the service was originally established to improve the availability of services for children in the South-West of England.

Nevertheless, having received expert advice, the inquiry report concluded that for open-heart surgery on children aged under one:

> between 1988 and 1994 the mortality rate at Bristol was roughly double that elsewhere in five out of seven years. This mortality rate failed to follow the overall downward trend over time which can be seen in other centres ... The mortality rate over the period 1991 1994 was probably double the rate in England at the time for children under 1, and even higher for children under 30 days.
>
> (Kennedy 2001; Summary, para 26, 5)

Put differently, this suggests that in the four years between 1991 and 1995 around 30 to 35 five more deaths of children under one occurred at Bristol than would have been expected had its mortality rate matched the national average.

The inquiry noted that some clinicians attributed the higher mortality rate at Bristol to the case mix, in other words, suggesting that they were dealing with more difficult cases. This is a potentially important point and an issue that needs to be considered when data between locations is compared. However, the inquiry report rejected this interpretation. Instead, it focused on failures within the system, paying particular attention to the relationship between the patient and the health care professional.

Culture and communication

A chapter of the inquiry report dealing with this relationship provides the following summary of the messages from Bristol:

> The service in Bristol was based on a paternalistic approach to families and to the care and support they needed;
>
> The culture in Bristol was not one which encouraged openness and honesty in the exchange of information between and amongst healthcare professionals and between them and families;
>
> Support and counselling particularly at the time of bereavement did not have a sufficiently high priority;

Communication was too often left by senior clinicians to nurses or junior doctors because it was time consuming and could be emotionally taxing.

(Kennedy 2001: 280)

The inquiry drew a distinction between what it perceived to be the situation in primary care and that which prevailed in the hospital sector. The report suggests that patients are more likely to experience being treated as equal partners by their GP, but when entering hospital find themselves confronted by 'old-style paternalistic attitudes' from some consultants (Kennedy 2001: 285)

The importance of trust in the relationship between professional experts and the public was referred to in Chapter 3, and the inquiry report considers steps judged necessary for trust to develop. The report argues that: 'the provision of adequate information is an essential prerequisite to the development of trust. It underpins the honesty between professional and patient' (Kennedy 2001: 287).

Several recommendations are made to increase the amount of information with which patients are provided. Support is given to a proposal made in the NHS Plan of 2000 that patients receive a copy of any letter written from one clinician to another. Going beyond this, it is recommended that patients are permitted to tape-record consultations, with facilities for this being provided by the NHS. The origins of this proposal lay in comments made to the inquiry by parents of very sick children who described how difficult it often was to recall details of what was said during highly stressful consultations. Examples were given where two parents found themselves having different recollections of the same discussions. Although, since April 2004, patients have been entitled to receive copies of letters written about them by one clinician to another, the right to record the consultation has not been introduced.

Alder Hey Inquiry

The concept of paternalism was also at the centre of the inquiry into the removal of body organs from deceased children at the Royal Liverpool Children's Hospital:

We set out to discover how so many parents were induced into thinking that they were burying their children intact when in fact the large majority were buried without their vital organs. In our search we discovered the long-standing widespread practice of organ retention without consent. The practice arose from a sense of paternalism on the part of the medical profession which served to conceal retention in the supposed best interest of the parents. Such practice was misconceived and was bound to cause upset and distress when, inevitably, it came to light.

(Redfern 2001: 444)

Unlike the situation at Bristol, what happened at Liverpool cannot be said to have influenced clinical outcomes. The issues involved children who had already died. But because of this, the matter was charged with intense emotional content. The inquiry report into Alder Hey Hospital reveals an immense accumulation of organs taken from the bodies of deceased or stillborn children. During various periods since the 1940s, 2128 hearts were collected together with 1564 stillbirths or pre-viable fetuses. A further 475 fetuses were retained at another location. Twenty-two body parts from 15 children included 13 post-natal heads and parts of heads from children from a few days old to 11 years of age. There were 22 heads from late premature/term fetuses. One child's whole body had been retained, separated in two containers: the body was in one and the head in the other. Other collections included 188 eyes and two optic nerves from 109 'specimens'. The inquiry report added, 'Perhaps the most disturbing specimen is that of the head of a boy aged 11 years'.

Informed consent

An issue providing the central focus for much of the inquiry report was 'informed consent'. Had parents knowingly consented to the removal of various organs from the bodies of their deceased children? In very many cases it was clear they had not. Parents described how they had been given little information, and that in any case this occurred at a hugely difficult and emotional time for them. Typical accounts are illustrated in the following examples:

> Not a lot that was said actually went in ... I was told it had to be done to check on the surgeon ... I signed the paper through tears and just wanted to grieve at home. I feel I was rushed into signing ... I feel that I should have been there to protect her. I do understand that these things need to be done but only with full permission and a full explanation.
>
> When they ask you to sign the form you are in so much turmoil you could sign your life away and would not know it.
>
> I wish they had explained things to us.

Presented with this kind of evidence, the inquiry into events at Alder Hey Hospital drew the following conclusion:

> We accept that for some clinicians it might be unpleasant to provide the detailed information necessary to obtain consent. However, their responsibility cannot be avoided. A practical test for the clinician in considering whether he has given full information is to question whether any significant detail not mentioned could have led to a different decision by the next of kin. If so then the test for fully informed consent will not have been met.
>
> (Redfern 369–70)

For both inquiry reports, Liverpool and Bristol, the issue of paternalism is intimately bound up with the notion of 'informed consent'. Interventions should not only proceed with consent but this consent must be 'informed'. However, if we try to understand these issues concerning the patient–practitioner relationship in isolation we fail to appreciate some of the contextual factors that help explain them.

Styles of decision making

Styles of decision making reflect the fact that different clinical and therapeutic settings demand different responses. In a discussion on providing information to patients, Coulter (2001) refers to this by describing three different styles of decision making:

- professional choice: the clinician decides and the patient consents
- shared decision making: information is shared with the patient and clinician coming to a decision together
- consumer choice: the clinician informs and the patient makes the decision.

Coulter suggests each may have its place in particular settings. It is relatively easy to think of examples where one or another might be more appropriate. What may be necessary in an emergency situation would not be appropriate for providing advice about contraception. But, in many cases, the appropriate category may not be self-evident. Judgements need to be made but how should these be informed? One view, expressed in an editorial in the *British Medical Journal*, is that: 'For doctors the trick will be to determine which patients want to be offered choice and which prefer a passive role' (British Medical Journal 1999).

This might be seen a simply moving paternalism a little bit further along; with the professional determining whether patients want to choose. The comment may be a little unfair, as these matters do involve difficult balances, but it illustrates a need to have some framework within which these dilemmas can be considered. As a part of this, the remainder of this chapter discusses the relationship between patients and professionals in terms of three dimensions or challenges to paternalism: the informed patient, the 'expert patient', and the patient as a customer.

The informed patient

Failures in communication about illness and treatment are the most frequent source of patient dissatisfaction (Coulter 2002). Lack of information was identified as a significant source of complaint in a survey of 2249 patients who had recently been discharged from hospitals in the UK (Coulter 2001). Fifty-nine per cent of those responding said they were not given enough say in decisions about treatment. In addition, 20 per cent said staff did not always treat them with respect and dignity and 29 per cent said that doctors sometimes talked about them as if they were not there (Coulter 2001). Coulter also notes that criticisms about experiences could differ between social groups and that: 'Desire for participation has been found to vary according to age, educational status, disease severity and cultural background' (Coulter 2001).

Inadequacies in the provision of information may not only limit the capacity of patients to make choices, it has implications for the level of involvement in managing a condition. For example, in a survey carried out by the Audit Commission, involving a national sample of 1400 people with diabetes, 40 per cent did not know if their HbAlc had been measured in the previous year (Raleigh and Clifford 2002).

Providing more comprehensive information to patients appears to have effects but these are not always as straightforward as might be expected. A large-scale review of randomized control trials into the role of 'decision aids' – or 'shared decision-making programmes' – found considerable variations in results between studies but the overall conclusion was that: 'decision aids do a better job than usual care in improving patients' knowledge about options, reducing their decisional conflict, and stimulating patients to take a more active role in decision making without increasing their anxiety' (O'Conner et al. 1999: 733).

Despite this, there appeared to be little effect on levels of patient satisfaction, and the impact on the actual decisions taken was variable. We need to look more closely at how information and decisions are being shared, if we are to isolate those factors that may be contributing to variable outcomes. One study in shared information that did this found no evidence that it altered patient choice.

Knowledge, information and status

The study, conducted in 13 Welsh maternity units, investigated the impact of information leaflets upon choices made by women. The leaflets were of a type commonly used in maternity departments but, in a result the authors describe as 'surprising', it was found that: 'the use of Informed Choice leaflets did not change the proportion of women who reported exercising informed choice, or components or consequences of informed choice, in maternity care' (O'Cathain et al. 2002: 324).

It is impossible to know why this might be so but it suggests that simply providing the information may be insufficient. Much can depend upon the context in which this is received. Of particular importance can be the character of the interaction with professionals. One recent study explored this by examining treatment choices made by women with menorrhagia, in six hospitals in South West England. Options available were: first, receiving surgical treatment (hysterectomy or endometrial ablation); second, receiving drug therapy; and third, having other possible interventions, including dilatation and curettage, and removal of the contraceptive coil.

The study included nearly nine hundred patients, randomly allocated to one of three groups. The first group received the existing, standard form of care; the second received an information pack; and the third received the information pack and a structured interview with a nurse. The study concluded that the receipt of additional information by two groups: 'helped the women form treatment preferences and these tended to be more conservative than those of the group that did not receive the information package'.

In other words, fewer women in the groups receiving the information package chose to have a hysterectomy than in the group receiving the standard care.

However, the difference was most marked for the group receiving an interview with a nurse in addition to the information package. Was this because it helped explain the information? Possibly; but the results suggest something more:

> The nurses' role was important in helping women to get what they wanted. Those who had the information without the interview knew what they wanted, but they seemed less able to communicate their preference to the gynaecologist.
>
> (Kennedy *et al.* 2002: 21).

Communication and hierarchy

The need to improve the communication skills of health professionals was recognized by the Bristol Inquiry report:

> Education in communication skills must be an essential part of the education of all healthcare professionals. Communication skills include the ability to engage with patients on an emotional level, to listen, to assess how much information a patient wants to know, and to convey information with clarity and sympathy.
>
> (Kennedy, 2001: 445)

Responding to the Inquiry report, the Department of Health agreed: 'more emphasis should be placed upon the non-clinical aspects of care, such as communication skills, in the education, training and development of those working within the NHS' (Department of Health 2002).

Welcome though this may be, attention must be given to the hierarchical relationships within which communication takes place. However much the interaction between a patient and a professional can appear to be a one-to-one relationship, in reality it is shaped by wider relationships surrounding it. Improving ways in which information is communicated to patients is important, but this may need to be accompanied by giving greater support to patients in making their views known.

Communicating uncertainty

Circumstances in which the communication of information can raise greatest difficulties are those in which prognosis is poor but uncertain. A very early study on this topic, conducted in the United States, looked at the experiences of 14 families with a child who had contracted paralytic poliomyelitis. The results showed that, in the early stages, it was very difficult to make a definite prognosis of likely impairment:

> During this initial period of the child's hospitalization, the physician is hardly ever able to tell the parents anything definite about the child's prospects of regaining lost muscular function ... To the parents' insistent question 'How

will he come out of it?', the invariable response of treatment personnel was that they did not know and that only time would tell.

(Davis 1960)

As the doctors were able to form more definite judgements, a question examined by the study was how this information was communicated to parents:

On the basis of intensive and repeated interviewing of the parents over the two year period, the answer to these questions is that, except for one case in which the muscle check pointed clearly to full recovery, the parents were neither told nor explicitly prepared by the treatment personnel to expect an outcome significantly different from that which they understandably hoped for, namely, a complete and natural recovery for the child. This does not imply that the doctors issued falsely optimistic progress or that, through indirection or other subtleties, they sought to encourage the parents to expect more by way of recovery than was possible. Rather, what typically transpired was that the parents were kept in the dark. The doctors' answers to their questions were couched for the most part in such hedging, evasive, or unintelligibly technical terms as to cause them, from many such contacts, to expect a more favourable recovery than could be justified by the facts then known. As one treatment-staff member put it, 'We try not to tell them too much. It's better if they find out for themselves in a natural sort of way.'

(Davis 1960: 156)

Echoes of the message of this older study recur in the inquiries into events at Alder Hey and Bristol. The latter report recounts:

We heard that much of the current information for patients about treatment is out of date, or of poor quality. Criticism was particularly levelled at infor-mation which is excessively optimistic, and that which has a tendency to downplay, or omit mention of, side effects, risks, uncertainties and con-troversies. We would add that too often the information given to patients seeks to encourage compliance with what is proposed, rather than to engage patients with the choices which are theirs to make, and thereby empower them.

(Kennedy 2001: 287–8)

As a contrast, the Inquiry reports comments made by a mother describing a neurologist who had treated her daughter:

'Although what he had to tell us was so bleak, we appreciated his very direct approach. We wanted the truth as he saw it, and he respected our wish to be fully informed.' She went on to express her appreciation also of her daughter's cardiologist's ability to respond in '. . . a normal, human way . . .' and the nurses' willingness to '. . . share part of themselves on a human mother-to-mother level.'

(Kennedy 2001: 282)

Comments by other parents of sick children made to the Inquiry emphasized similar concerns: 'I think you need to know. It hurts ... It hurts to hear it, but you need to know the truth. I do not want to be told everything is going to be jolly and fine. It is a fact of life ... You do not want people to be cruel to you but you need honesty in a situation like that' (Kennedy 2001: 282).

Improving communication skills is important, but unlikely to be sufficient unless the character of the relationship between professional and patient is also considered. In particular, this means taking account of the mutual exchange of knowledge, recognizing that the relationship is not merely about how information is disseminated by the professional. It also involves making effective use of the expertise of the patient or parent, and acknowledging the continuing importance of emotions.

The expert patient

In 2001 the Chief Medical Officer issued a publication on chronic illness, urging a shift towards recognizing the role patients can play in its management (*The Expert Patient*). This idea, drawn from approaches developed in the United States, emphasizes the knowledge that patients themselves possess:

> The second half of the 20th Century and the beginning of the new century has been a period in which many more people have lived into their seventies, eighties and beyond. This greater longevity has brought with it an increased burden of heart disease, stroke, cancer, arthritis, diabetes mellitus, mental illness, asthma and other conditions. As a result, the predominant disease pattern in England, and most other developed countries, is one of chronic or long-term illness rather than acute disease.
>
> (p. 4)
>
> Research and practical experience in North America and Britain are showing that today's patients with chronic diseases need not be mere recipients of care. They can become key decision-makers in the treatment process. By ensuring that knowledge of their condition is developed to a point where they are empowered to take some responsibility for its management and work in partnership with their health and social care providers, patients can be given greater control over their lives. Self-management programmes can be specifically designed to reduce the severity of symptoms and improve confidence, resourcefulness and self-efficacy.
>
> (Department of Health 2001: 5)

Several studies are referred to in the report to support the efficacy of this approach, but it is difficult to envisage real movement in this direction within traditional patient–professional relationships. Reviewing research in this field, Coulter reports examples pointing to the implications that a more active role for patients may have:

Patients with hypertension benefit if they are allowed to adopt an active rather than a passive role in treatment, patients with breast cancer suffer less depression and anxiety if they are treated by doctors who adopt a participative consultation style, and patients who are more actively involved in discussions about the management of their diabetes achieve better blood sugar control. Patients whose doctors are ignorant of their values and preferences may receive treatment that is inappropriate to their needs.

(Coulter *et al.* 1999)

In light of this, it may be significant to note results from a study conducted in the United States in the 1980s that found doctors gave their patients an average of 18 seconds to give their accounts before interrupting them and steering the discussion towards a medical agenda they regarded as appropriate (Beckman and Frankel 1984).

In a study of British nurses, Clark (1981) found that during a two-hour period student nurses would spend on average 21.7 minutes in conversation with patients, compared to 16.2 minutes spent by trained nurses. The average length of each conversation was 2 minutes and 1.4 minutes respectively. One possible factor is that qualified nurses have more duties to perform, but the role of established routines may also be important: 'Nurse–patient conversations tend to be short, often (but not always) occur in relation to tasks and, in content, are almost exclusively restricted to technical rather than emotional matters' (Clark 1981: 14).

Nor is it simply a matter of short consultations. It is also apparent that length of consultation can be influenced by social factors unconnected to the condition or diagnosis. One study in the 1970s, based on tape recordings of 92 patient consultations with GPs, found the average length of consultations with middle-class patients was 6.2 minutes, compared to an average of 4.7 minutes received by working-class patients. Working-class patients had on average three symptoms but with an average of 2.8 problems being discussed during their consultations. In contrast, with an average of 2.2 symptoms, middle-class patients were able to discuss an average of 4.1 problems (Cartwright and O'Brien 1976).

Differences of this kind no doubt contributed to the conclusion drawn by Cartwright (1983) in a later review: 'One finding from a number of studies is that working class people differ little from middle class in their desire for information but the middle class are more successful in obtaining it' (p. 128).

Social class has long been noted as a significant factor influencing the quality of patient–professional interactions, perhaps most obviously in the contrast between private practice and the NHS. In 1958 Sir Thomas Holmes Sellors, a leading consultant, addressing a commission established to enquire into doctors' pay, stated bluntly: 'To put it rather unofficially ... to put it rather crudely, in an (NHS) out-patients session the patient listens to the doctor, whereas in a private practice, the consultant listens to the patients' (Cited in Ferris 1967: 34).

Mulcahy (2003) concludes from an analysis of NHS complaints data that patients and doctors frequently focus on different aspects. Whereas doctors often emphasized technical matters, communication and the attitude of staff was given priority by many patients. It is suggested that: 'The high incidence of complaints relating to communication does not necessarily result from inattentiveness or insensitivity but from a more fundamental disagreement about the nature of illness' (Mulcahy 2003: 88).

Treating patients as experts in their own right requires a shift in the relationship between them and professionals. Private practice may, to some degree, represent a recreation of older relationships where patients really were customers. As many urge, is this the model to which we should be looking?

Consumerism and the patient as 'customer'

In a speech prepared for the 2001 British Trades Union Congress, but not delivered because of the terrorist outrages in New York, the Prime Minister, Tony Blair, pressed for 'changes in the way we treat the patient as a customer. More choice for the pupil, patient or customer and the ability if provision is poor, to have an alternative provider' (TUC website, 13 Sep 2001).

Tony Blair is one of the latest politicians to focus on this issue, a trend that has been apparent since the 1980s at least, as Pollitt (1987) observed:

'Consumerism' has become an officially approved fashion. In hospitals, schools, housing schemes, advice and information services and many other aspects of public administration managers are being exhorted to pay more attention to consumer wishes, offer consumers wider choice, and develop techniques for 'marketing' their particular service.

(Pollitt 1987: 43)

The early application of 'consumerism' to contexts such as health care was discussed by the sociologist Margaret Stacey in the 1970s. She noted a tendency to apply to the NHS ways of thinking about work and organizations developed in economic and industrial spheres, and the influence of the growth of the consumer movement. However, Stacey points out significant differences. In particular: 'The important distinction in health is that this is a service industry which does things *to* people rather than *for* people'.

She was not implying that this means patients are passive recipients of a service. Instead, the fact that something is being done to them, rather than for them, means they are more likely to seek engagement: 'the health service is better thought of as a process of more or less prolonged interaction between the minds and bodies of the patients and the health care workers' (Stacey 1976).

One field of health care that provides a striking example of the consequences of paying attention to doing things to people rather than for people is childbirth. Here there has been long-standing controversy over the extent to which women should have their decisions circumscribed by doctors, but it can be a mistake to see this as a straightforward conflict between professionals and patients. This can be illustrated by considering developments in the management of pain during labour.

Choices in childbirth

Roy Porter describes the first use of chloroform for a woman in labour, administered by James Young Simpson, professor of surgery in Edinburgh, who discovered its anaesthetic properties in 1831. In 1853 Queen Victoria received chloroform from her doctor John Snow (who later became better known for is work in public health) during the birth of her son, Prince Leopold. The Queen later described the experience in her diary: 'The effect was soothing, quieting and delightful beyond measure.'

However, others were not so positive, with *The Lancet* objecting: 'In no case could it be justifiable to administer chloroform in perfectly normal labour.' Others argued on religious grounds, referring to biblical references that women should experience pain during birth (Porter 1997: 367–8). Since then, medical interventions during childbirth have remained controversial, a recent example being the rising rates of caesarean births. In 1970s Britain around 5 per cent of all births were by caesarean delivery, a rate that had risen to 13 per cent by 1992. This was still considerably below the rate of 24 per cent in the US in the mid-1980s (Foster 1995: 40–1). Foster reports a survey of 135 British obstetricians in 1983, in which they were asked to explain the rising rate of caesareans. Three particular causes were suggested.

Most frequently mentioned (by 41 per cent of the obstetricians) was the fact that responses to dealing with breech deliveries had changed, with a caesarean being automatically used in many cases. Second in importance, referred to by 28 per cent, was a fear of litigation. In the words of one of the doctors: 'should I produce a brain-damaged baby by forceps delivery in 1983, that child can accuse me of negligence in a court of law until 2004 ... I like to think it does not unduly influence my clinical judgement ...' (Francome 1986: 101, cited in Foster 1995: 41).

The third most commonly mentioned reason was the increase in fetal monitoring, referred to by 25 per cent of the obstetricians. Many remained unconvinced that these explanations provided adequate justification for the increasing rate. For instance, a study published in *The Lancet* of 50 caesareans prompted by fetal distress concluded that one-third may have been unnecessary (Barrett *et al.* 1990. Other studies comparing women who had received caesarean deliveries and those who had delivered vaginally found the former experienced higher rates and longer lasting depression, took longer to feel close to their infants, as well as having quite high rates of wound infection (reported in Foster 1995). Most critics acknowledge the benefits of caesarean delivery in certain circumstances but argue that too often it was being used inappropriately. The medical profession was seen as using too readily surgical procedures available to it, even though these might interfere with the emotional and psychological experience of childbirth. From this perspective, women's choice was being constrained and directed by the inappropriate use of professional authority and expertise.

These concerns prompted a considerable movement intended to give women a greater say in arrangements for childbirth. However, the rate of caesarean deliveries has continued to rise. A report commissioned by the National Institute of

Clinical Excellence, established to provide advice on good clinical practice, reviewed the reasons for which caesareans were performed, finding that:

> Although CS rates have increased over the last ten to fifteen years, the four major clinical determinants of the CS rate have not changed. These remain fetal compromise (22 per cent), 'failure to progress' in labour (20 per cent), repeat CS (14 per cent) and breech (11 per cent). The fifth most common reason given for performing a CS has changed and is now reported to be 'maternal request' (7 per cent).
>
> (National Institute of Clinical Excellence, 2004b: 1)

The report goes on to give considerable attention to the question of whether mothers should be able to request a caesarean in the absence of clinical conditions indicating its use. This includes a review of evidence on reasons why this option is requested in such circumstance:

> The rates of preference for CS expressed by the women that were surveyed during pregnancy in UK, Australia and Sweden range from 6 per cent–8 per cent. Within these studies there was a consistent relationship between women's preference for CS and either previous CS, previous negative birth experience, a complication in the current pregnancy or a fear of giving birth.
>
> (National Institute of Clinical Excellence 2004b: 37)

The report notes that obstetricians estimate that they agree to perform a CS for about half of the requests they receive, but concludes with the following recommendations:

> Maternal request is not on its own an indication for CS and specific reasons for the request should be explored, discussed and recorded.
>
> When a woman requests a CS in the absence of an identifiable reason, the overall benefits and risks of CS compared with vaginal birth should be discussed and recorded.
>
> When a woman requests a CS because she has a fear of childbirth, she should be offered counselling (such as cognitive behavioural therapy) to help her to address her fears in a supportive manner, because this results in reduced fear of pain in labour and shorter labour.
>
> An individual clinician has the right to decline a request for CS in the absence of an identifiable reason. However, the woman's decision should be respected and she should be offered referral for a second opinion.
>
> (National Institute for Clinical Excellence, 2004b: 38)

Again, choice becomes a difficult concept. In this case because it involves a procedure that is judged clinically unnecessary, has some risks, and costs around £1275 more per birth than a vaginal delivery. As with the MMR vaccine, the option of using a private service may be available to some but this is not the main focus for this discussion. In a state-provided health care system there are genuine difficulties in applying apparently sensible ideas about the benefits of extending choice. Professionals tend to find themselves dealing with the tensions that can arise, and are required to find ways of reconciling different kinds of knowledge, values, emotions and cultural traditions.

Barriers to patient choice

One reason why some professionals may find it difficult to encourage patient choice is they feel they are working in an institutional environment unable to respond flexibly and meet every individual request. Pressures to complete tasks may inhibit scope for effective communication. A doctor nominated by the Royal College of Psychiatrists to examine accounts of hundreds of patients who reported negative experiences they believed were associated with taking antidepressants, expressed concern about how it had been prescribed. The patients had contacted the BBC programme, Panorama, after it had reported on similar cases:

> DR ALFRED WHITE (Royal College of Psychiatrists): The first impression was the vast majority of the people shouldn't have been on the drug in the first place. There were hardly any, if any, that I saw where I felt convinced that they had an illness which would be appropriate. It's an extremely good anti-depressant, extremely useful drug for the right illness, can be lifesaving. And if you give it to anybody with life problems then you're going to over prescribe it and you're going to cause problems as well as solving them.
>
> SHELLEY JOFREY (Presenter): Is it any wonder if it's over prescribed though? More than a third of our respondents said they were put on Seroxat after just five or ten minutes with their often hard-pressed doctors. That surely isn't long enough to diagnose depression and prescribe a drug like Seroxat?
>
> DR JIM KENNEDY (Royal College of General Practitioners): Certainly it is good practice to spend an appropriate amount of time on diagnosing and monitoring depression. It is probably not appropriate to spend such a short time as five or so minutes on this kind of problem.
>
> (BBC 2003)

Institutional failures on a wider scale can also occur. They can also cause real damage, creating problems well beyond those of lack of time. In the 1960s and 1970s a series of investigations were held into conditions in long-stay NHS hospitals, prompted by allegations of neglect and abuse. There have been enormous changes since then but features of the institutional climate, identified in a review of the inquiry reports, may continue to be relevant. Martin (1984) notes that several organizational failings were common in many of the cases examined, for example: 'Inquiry after inquiry showed that the worst wards were hardly ever visited by consultants, and not always by junior medical staff' (Martin 1984: 81).

Furthermore: 'Almost always it seems to have been known at "grass roots" level that certain wards, and indeed certain individuals, were "bad" ... At higher levels it also seems quite possible for staffs at Area, Regional or even National level to know of unsatisfactory conditions, but for no effective action to have been taken' (Martin 1984: 84–5).

However, of greatest relevance here is the capacity for individual and organizational failings to coalesce to create a 'corruption of care':

> An important feature of the regimes revealed by the inquiries has been what can be termed the corruption of care. By this is meant the fact that the primary aims of care – the cure or alleviation of suffering – have become subordinate to what are essentially secondary aims such as the creation and presentation of order, quiet and cleanliness. Of course these have their place, but as means to ends and not ends in themselves.
>
> (Martin 1984: 86–7)

No direct comparison is intended between events at Bristol and Alder Hey and those occurring in some of the long-stay hospitals three decades ago. The point being made is a different one. Serious thought needs to be given to the extent to which a 'customer' relationship is the right response for avoiding both the 'corruption of care' and paternalism. Rather than seeking to adopt a customer-based model, having its roots in commercial contexts, there may be greater value in reflecting on the alternative approach urged by Stacey. This might accord more closely with experiences of patients and carers. One point noted by the Bristol Inquiry was that, as well as wanting more information, a strong message from parents was the desire to be treated with respect and honesty. In the words of one mother:

> You cannot trust people if you do not think they are being honest, even if they are being nice. Once you think that they might not say the thing as it is, then you can never believe quite – there is no working relationship from that point on.
>
> (Kennedy 2001: 282)

Recognizing that patients and professionals need to establish a 'working relationship' demands we think beyond the rather simplistic and service model of the patient as customer. This is a theme that has been developed by former GP, Julian Tudor Hart, who suggests that the patient and professional should be regarded as 'co-workers'. To support this approach, he refers to one study, conducted in the 1970s, which suggested that patients contribute at least 85 per cent of the information on which a diagnosis is based (Hart 1975).

Hart is critical of consumer-based models, as he regards the interaction between the patient and professional as requiring a quite different relationship:

> In effective consultations, patients don't behave like consumers ... When doctors and patients consult with optimal efficiency, they become co-producers. In essence, consultations are not units of consumption, but units of production. Something has been created at the end of the consultation, which was not present at the beginning: more and better understanding of patients'

problems, of possible solutions, and of the personal circumstances in which these must be applied, leading to health gain as a social product as well as a personal good.

(Hart 1998: 9)

This approach recognizes that patients have lives and contexts beyond the specific problem that brings them into contact with a health professional. It also provides a suitable point at which to shift the focus of the book, from the patient–professional relationship to wider aspects of the social distribution of health. Unless interactions between patient and professional take account of these factors they are unlikely to develop in ways that allow a true exchange of knowledge. The next four chapters explore different aspects of the social distribution of health, before Chapter 10 reconnects this with the earlier themes by considering ways in which health care services are used unequally by different social groups.

Part 2

Health care and the social distribution of illness

6
Society, health and health care

Despite considerable differences in the arguments of writers who challenged the positive image of modern medicine, such as Ivan Illich and Irving Zola, a common objection is that medicine becomes inappropriately involved in personal problems and difficulties with living. The 'medicalizing of everyday life' is seen as an undesirable retreat from dealing with the moral and emotional challenges of what it means to be human.

Others take a different line, including some such as Cornwell, who also use the term 'medicalization'. Cornwell is less negative about the role of medicine, regarding it as an important source of intervention in problems that cause real pain and suffering. From this perspective, the problem can be one of not too much medical intervention but, for some social groups at least, too little. This question is addressed in Chapter 10, in a discussion on inequalities in access to health care.

How can the contribution made by medicine to our health be reliably assessed? This is a controversial area, and one way of approaching it is to begin with a short historical example on the decline of infectious diseases. This illustrates the emerging dominance of clinical medicine, while providing an opportunity to consider other branches, particularly those of public health medicine, and its shorter-lived cousin, social medicine. Comparisons between these different branches of medicine offer a way of considering alternatives to the traditional focus of clinical medicine upon the individual patient and the disease.

This theme develops in later parts of the chapter to a discussion on the extent to which health professionals can or should be involved in addressing the wider context of patients' lives. As a contrast to the dominant focus on Western medicine, this includes some examples drawn from the Cuban health care system.

A social history of infection

At different points in history, various diseases have provided a focus for social, political and emotional attention. Writing about cholera in the nineteenth century, the social historian Asa Briggs describes it as:

> a disease of society in the most profound sense. Whenever cholera threatened European countries it quickened social apprehensions. Wherever it appeared,

it tested the efficiency and resilience of local administrative structures. It exposed relentlessly political, social, and moral shortcomings. It prompted rumours, suspicions, and, at times, violent social conflicts.

(Briggs 1961)

Cholera killed 32,000 people in Britain in 1832. Sixteen years later twice as many died. In 1841, average life expectancy at birth was just 26.6 years in Manchester and 28.1 in Liverpool. Much of this was due to appallingly high death rates among infants. Of the total of 350,000 deaths in 1842, 140,000 were of children under five years of age (Hunt 2004: 28–9). Faced with death on such a scale, the nineteenth century saw considerable debate around the causes of infectious diseases such as cholera. In these debates different views emerged towards the roles played by the infectious agent itself, and the wider environment. The relative effect of each, in turn, has implications for judging the contribution that clinical treatments have made to the decline of infectious disease. In a noted analysis, Thomas McKeown argues that the decline in a wide range of infectious diseases over the past 150 years is largely a consequence of improved nutrition and reduced overcrowding. The contribution made by medicine is not denied but judged relatively minor in comparison to these improvements: 'the health of man is determined essentially by his behaviour, his food and the nature of the world around him, and is only marginally influenced by personal medical care' (McKeown 1979).

Competing theories

If we place ourselves for a moment in the debates of the mid-nineteenth century, we hear strongly competing accounts of the causes of infectious diseases. On one side, proponents of 'miasma theories'; on the other, advocates of 'contagion theories'. Miasma was described by Dr William Duncan, the Medical Officer of Health for Liverpool, as the 'vitiation [i.e. impairment] of the atmosphere of towns'. He saw urban overcrowding, together with the waste it generated, as creating disease, causing air to become 'unfit for the purpose of respiration' (Quoted in Frazer 1950: 38). For most of the first half of the nineteenth century it was miasma theory, sometimes referred to as hygiene theory, which received endorsement.

The alternative theory of contagion, though not widely accepted, had a long lineage. In a verse written in 1530 about the 'French disease', the Veronese physician Fracastoro told of a shepherd, Syphilis, who having insulted Apollo was punished with a 'pestilence unknown', bringing 'foul sores' to his body. Fracastoro later developed the idea to explain contagious disease as the consequence of 'seeds' that could infect by contact (Porter 1999: 174–5).

Although this idea had continued to feature in ideas about disease, one objection was that it failed to explain how epidemics emerged in the first place. This weakness helped support the continuing influence of miasma theories, although developments in bacteriology by the later nineteenth century were to alter this. By 1878, proposing what became known as 'germ theory', Louis Pasteur was arguing that micro-organisms were responsible for disease. Four years later Robert Koch identified *Mycobacterium tuberculosis* as being responsible for tuberculosis, and in the following year revealed the cause of cholera to lie with *Vibrio cholera*. Bacteriology was not always capable of producing effective treatments but, as Roy Porter remarks, 'in the twenty-one golden years between 1879 and 1900 the micro-organisms responsible for major diseases were being discovered at the phenomenal rate of one per year' (Porter 1999: 442).

Not all scientists at the time supported this focus. Critics continued to emphasize the role of the environment, challenging the claim that a single bacillus could cause disease. These were matters on which intense views were held. One opponent of contagion theory went to quite amazing lengths to demonstrate its alleged shortcomings. During a cholera outbreak in Hamburg in 1892, Max von Pettenkofer asked Robert Koch to send him a flask of *Vibrio cholera*, which he then drank. No doubt he felt vindicated as a bout of diarrhoea appears to have been the only ill effect (Baldwin 1999: 167; Porter 1999: 437).

Contagion theorists remained unconvinced. Bacteriology grew in influence, though its proponents accepted that the environment could be important for determining *how* infection spread. Its growth in influence can perhaps be explained largely by the fact that bacteriology proved capable of explaining routes of disease transmission, generating results from laboratory-based research that could not be achieved by alternative accounts.

Thomas McKeown and the 'limits of medicine'

One of the infectious diseases discussed by McKeown is respiratory tuberculosis, for which he regards medicine's main contribution as being the introduction of streptomycin in 1948. If we assume that without streptomycin, mortality rates from tuberculosis would have continued at the same rate as from 1921 to 1946, then the drug can be judged as having cut death rates by 51 per cent between 1947 and 1971. By any account, this is a considerable achievement. As Porter observes: 'Tuberculosis had been steadily declining over the previous century; antibiotics delivered the final blow' (Porter 1999: 458).

McKeown attributes the whole of this decline to the drugs, rather than the BCG vaccine introduced soon afterwards, on the grounds that reductions of a similar scale were achieved in other countries without a vaccination programme. For example, the Netherlands had no national BCG programme yet showed the lowest death rates from respiratory tuberculosis for any European country in 1957–9 and 1967–9 (McKeown 1979: 92–4).

However, McKeown's main argument is that if we consider medicine's contribution in the context of the whole period from 1848 (when causes of death were first recorded) to 1971, then it can claim to have achieved just 3.2 per cent of the total reduction. McKeown concludes:

> Effective clinical intervention came late in the history of the disease, and over the whole period of its decline the effect was small in relation to that of other influences. But although the problems presented by tuberculosis in the mid

twentieth century were smaller than those in the early nineteenth, it was still a common and often fatal disease with a high level of associated morbidity. In two of its forms, tuberculosis meningitis and miliary tuberculosis, it was invariably fatal. The challenge to medical science and practice was to increase the rate of decline of mortality and, if possible, finally remove the threat of the disease which had been a leading cause of infectious deaths for nearly two centuries. In this it was outstandingly successful, and it would be as unreasonable to underestimate this achievement as to overlook the fact that it was preceded, and probably necessarily preceded, by modification of the conditions – low resistance from malnutrition and heavy exposure from overcrowding – which had made tuberculosis so formidable.

(McKeown 1979: 95–6)

It is important to stress again that McKeown is not dismissing the contribution of medicine. What he argues is that it was only able to achieve this because of the prior improvements, gained as a consequence of better nutrition and reduced overcrowding. Once these had been achieved, further gains require different interventions. Viewed from the perspective of mortality rates of the 1940s rather than the 1840s, the effect of pharmacological intervention was substantial.

McKeown's approach parallels that of Max von Pettenkofer, even though he employs statistical data rather than a more direct empirical test. The essential argument is that, rather than concentrate on the bacteriological agent, we should pay more attention to the fact that a healthy body provides the best defence against disease. This is why McKeown argues that improved nutrition is the biggest single factor contributing to the decline in infectious disease in the nineteenth century: 'we have concentrated on specific measures such as vaccination and environmental improvement without sufficient regard for the predominant part played by nutritional state' (McKeown 1979: 62–3).

Individual health and public health

This, though, is not the only alternative to a bacteriological emphasis. McKeown stresses the importance of nutrition and overcrowding, but others point to the role of different environmental factors. One historical account of this period describes two broad camps, in terms of 'sanitationist anti-vaccinators' and 'holistic anti-vaccinators' (Baldwin 1999: 288). An emphasis upon hygiene was fundamental for each, but the latter saw improvements coming through self-control and healthier lifestyles rather than better homes and drains. A corollary was that individual choice was seen as more important than collective action for remedying risks to health.

McKeown's analysis does not fall neatly into one or other of these positions and, to some extent, may be seen to straddle them. However, other interpretations of the historical evidence have drawn different conclusions. One example is found in the work of another historian, Simon Szreter, who identifies clean water as the single biggest contributing factor (Szreter 2001). Agreeing with McKeown's conclusion that medicine played a relatively minor role, Szreter does not support his assessment that the removal of malnutrition and overcrowding were the main factors. Pointing out that the greatest decline in mortality occurred from the 1870s, Szreter argues that the most significant factor was likely to have been new statutory responsibilities on local authorities to supply clean water, introduced in 1872. Szreter concludes that his account:

> indicates a primary role for those public health measures which combated the early nineteenth-century upsurge of diseases directly resulting from the defective and insanitary urban and domestic environments created in the course of industrialisation.
>
> (Szreter 2001: 226)

It would be a mistake to regard this as a matter of purely historical interest. Szreter's argument is intended to challenge what he regards as a major flaw in McKeown's account; that it, 'minimalised the role of directed human agency'. McKeown saw rises in the standard of living as being the major factor leading to improved nutrition and thereby reducing levels of disease, and in that sense regards economic growth, not public policy measures, as the prime determinant. Szreter believes this is wrong:

> the public health movement working through local government, rather than nutritional improvements through rising living standards, should be seen as the true moving force behind the decline of mortality in this period (217) ... there is a sound prima facie case to be answered that the decline in mortality, which began to be noticeable in the national aggregate statistics in the 1870s, was due more to the eventual successes of the politically and ideologically negotiated movement for public health than to any other positively identifiable factor.
>
> (Szreter 2001: 225)

If it is assumed that economic growth is the main engine of social progress, and that its benefits will more or less automatically 'trickle down' though society, then the role of politics and social movements may be judged of little importance. If, on the other hand, Szreter is right to emphasize the impact of public health measures, then these spheres of activity become vitally important. It is unnecessary here to evaluate the historical arguments in any greater detail but it is important to note the distinction between approaches that assume an almost direct link between economic growth and health status, and those that see the relationship as mediated by political action. In the nineteenth century these issues came to the fore in concerns surrounding the spread of infectious disease. Today, chronic illness has to a considerable extent taken its place as a dominant cause of suffering. Relevant to both has been the unequal distribution of disease across society, an aspect that provides the main focus for later chapters.

Clinical medicine in the late twentieth century

Before proceeding to these issues, we need to consider a possibility that flows from McKeown's analysis: that the relative contribution of medicine has increased as other factors have led to an absolute decline in rates of infection. It might be argued that over a period of 120 years the role of medicine has been marginal but its relative contribution has increased as other causes have been conquered. An attempt to update McKeown's analysis has been made by Bunker (1995/2001) from a position broadly sympathetic to the role of medicine, who argues that, whereas McKeown examined data up to 1971: 'The quarter century that followed has seen an explosion of new medical treatments, many of which have been shown in clinical trials and meta-analysis to result in considerable improvements in health' (Bunker 2001: 234).

Bunker's analysis can be illustrated with one example, in which he draws on US data for medical interventions in heart disease (Goldman and Cook 1984). This suggested that 40 per cent of the decline in cardiac death rates between 1968 and 1976 could be attributed to coronary care units, treatment of hypertension, and medical and surgical treatment of ischaemic heart disease. A wide range of similar data is combined by Bunker to support the conclusion:

> All told, we estimated that together, clinical preventative and curative services can be credited with about five of the 30 years increased life-expectancy gained in the United States and in Great Britain during this century, i.e. 17 per cent or 18 per cent. This is certainly a good deal more than McKeown was able to identify 24 years ago, but still a relatively small contribution. To place a five year change in life-expectancy in perspective, however, it may be useful to consider that a gain of five years in life expectancy is roughly equivalent to the loss in life-expectancy that an individual suffers by smoking a pack a day starting at age 20; and it is roughly equivalent to the difference in life-expectancy between the top grade and unskilled workers in the Whitehall study of British civil servants.
>
> (Bunker 2001: 235)

Bunker acknowledges that the methods of calculation used in this study are 'less than precise, they are approximations extrapolated from secondary sources'. Other researchers have approached the same type of question using different methods. One study, using medical expertise, sought to identify the proportion of deaths that could be avoided with the provision of good medical treatment. Between five and 15 per cent of all deaths were deemed to be wholly treatable, and in that sense potentially avoidable. However, a larger proportion of deaths were assessed as being attributable to social and economic factors (Mackenbach, Bouvier-Colle and Jougla 1990).

With so many potential factors involved, a definitive assessment of medicine's contribution to improved health is unlikely to be agreed. And mortality rates, of course, are not the only relevant indicator of success. If medical interventions can improve the quality of our finite lives, most of us would probably want the treatment. On balance, it appears reasonable to conclude that the role of clinical medicine has become more significant today than during the much longer historical period considered by McKeown.

However, this assessment needs to be considered alongside the debates reviewed in Chapter 4, around the alleged inappropriate extension of medicine into 'everyday life'. Can these claims be reconciled? If medicine has succeeded in playing an increasingly beneficial role in banishing illness, has this been at the expense of allowing it to claim a role in areas of life where it has no place?

One way of considering this question – as with the history of infection – is to explore the social factors that may be implicated in the cause of disease, and then consider how these are explained and understood. An interesting historical pointer to this question is provided by what became known as 'social medicine'.

Social medicine and psychosocial medicine

During the 1930s, in Britain and elsewhere, the attention of many researchers, professionals and others was seized by the apparent relationship between health status and social and economic conditions of the time:

> The convergence upon an idea of social medicine was based upon the inter-war experience with the social and economic roots of ill health. For them, the medicine of the future would have to tackle chronic illness, whose roots lay in poverty, unemployment, bad housing, and occupational conditions.
>
> (Figlio 1987: 78)

What distinguished social medicine from clinical and other forms of medicine was described by the professor of Public Health and Social Medicine at the University of Edinburgh, F.A.E. Crew, in 1944:

> Social medicine is medical science in relation to groups of human beings ... It is not merely or mainly concerned with the prevention and elimination of sickness, but is concerned also and especially with the study of all social agencies which promote or impair the fullest realization of biologically and socially valuable human capacities. It includes the application to problems of health and disease of sociological concepts and methods.
>
> (Cited in Webster 1986)

The first Professor of Social Medicine in Britain, John Ryle at Oxford, believed the traditional focus of public health, on sanitation and water supply, needed to be expanded to embrace: 'the whole of the economic, nutritional, occupational, educational, and psychological opportunity or experience of the individual or the community' (Porter 1999: 643–4).

Several studies conducted during the inter-war years found increasing rates of non-infective chronic illnesses, pointing towards problems lying: 'within a population as a social group, rather than towards an increase in the more usual causal agents of disease' (Figlio 1987: 79).

Social medicine, work and health

The argument can be illustrated with one example, a study of rheumatic heart disease by J.N. Morris and Richard Titmuss, published in 1944. This pointed to the negative consequences of joblessness on morbidity, even where this did not lead to death, and also indicated these consequences were not easily removed:

> These results suggest that unemployment – or enforced leisure – led to a reduction in ulcer *mortality*: the death rate fell in those boroughs most heavily affected by unemployment. But when unemployment declined, *after pronounced depression*, mortality rose sharply. A return to work – but perhaps very insecure re-employment – meant more ulcer deaths.

> The managerial revolution, speed-up in the factory and on the road, the fungus growth of examinations, the squeezing out of the small shop-keepers all assist in making up what Ryle calls 'the mental and physical fret and stress of civilized city life'.
>
> (Morris and Titmuss 1944: 843–5)

This issue had attracted interest as early as 1926, when the Medical Sociology Group of the British Medical Association examined problems arising from monotony and disaffection in the work place (Figlio 1987: 81). Later, the health of people certified 'incapable of work' became a focus of attention for the medical officer for the Department of Health for Scotland, James Halliday. Brought into contact with the issue through his role as a medical referee for national health insurance claims, Halliday noted a large increase in claims in the inter-war period. Many of these received vague diagnoses such as 'debility', prompting allegations of 'excess claiming' that were frequently associated with the suggestion that this was linked to the extension of insurance coverage to women:

> Government officials complained about labels like 'debility', while women's representatives argued that they expressed forms of ill-health not properly seen or understood before. Analysing many thousands of cases referred to him as a medical referee, Halliday rebuffed official scepticism in similar terms: the vague diagnostic categories on sickness certificates documented the gap between the presentation of ill-health and the medical understanding of that ill-health.
>
> (Figlio 1987: 84)

Halliday came to the conclusion that a very large proportion of diagnosed cases were 'psychosomatic' in origin. By this he meant that the physical symptoms were real, but prompted by emotional and psychological causes. The conditions he considered included rheumatism, gastritis, hypertension, peptic ulcers and many others. Halliday brought together his thinking in a book published in 1948, *Psychosocial Medicine: A Study of the Sick Society*. Although little known today, Halliday's interest in the psychosocial origins of illness resonates closely with emerging contemporary debates.

Contrasting interpretations can be placed on the value of the approach of social medicine. In a positive light, it can be viewed as giving recognition to the need for health practitioners to understand the whole person, and not just the physical manifestation of sickness or incapacity. More negatively, it can be regarded as yet another example of interventions by professionals into aspects of life lying beyond their competence. Porter, for example, suggests that social medicine was pioneered by: 'medical progressives, typically politically left-wing, impressed by the socialization of medicine in the USSR, and convinced that medical professionals knew best' (Porter 1999: 643).

These are difficult issues and the failure of social medicine to establish itself with anything like the influence secured by clinical medicine makes a reliable historical assessment difficult. To consider this argument, the following section briefly identifies issues arising from one context where a model with at least some elements akin to social medicine has been adopted.

Post-revolution health and health care in Cuba

Since the Cuban revolution of 1958 there have been stunning improvements in health status. Current WHO statistics show life expectancy among males of 74.7 years and 79.2 years for women. This compares very favourably with figures for the US: 74.3 years for males and 79.5 years for females. Although male infant mortality in Cuba is higher than in the US, 11 deaths per 100,000 compared to seven in the US, for females the figures are very similar (eight in Cuba and nine in the US).

Cuba has achieved rapid improvements in nutritional standards, identified by McKeown as the chief influence on declining mortality in nineteenth-century Britain, and also in public health measures, emphasized by Szreter (Sanders and Carver 1985: 161–4). Before the 1958 revolution, several studies revealed widespread under-nutrition. One reported that one-third of the population, and 60 per cent in rural areas, was undernourished. By 1969, a report by the UN Food and Agricultural Association estimated the average daily calorific intake to have reached the daily requirement of 2500k cal. This was accompanied by improvements in housing, sewage systems and piped water (Sanders and Carver 1985).

All these factors no doubt contributed to the enormous improvements in health status. That conventional indicators of health status, such as life expectancy and infant mortality rates, now put Cuba more or less on a par with the US, rather than other Latin American and Caribbean countries, is particularly significant when levels of spending are considered.

The US spends nearly double the proportion of GDP on health care than is spent in Cuba – 13.0 per cent compared to 6.8 per cent. A comparison of how money is spent and the form of health care provision reveal some notable differences between the Cuban health care system and the model adopted in US.

Prior to the revolution, medical care was available only to those able to pay for it, and most services were concentrated in the capital, Havana. Despite the emigration of nearly half the country's doctors between the revolution and 1962, intense recruitment and training meant that by the early 1970s: 'the ratio of doctors to population in Cuba resembled that of the United States and surpassed that of all other Latin American Countries' (Waitzkin 1991: 265).

Substantial emphasis was placed upon the development of primary health care. New facilities were developed, with each province having a regional hospital supported by a network of clinics. Results have been impressive. For example, 80 per cent of all Cuban children were immunized against poliomyelitis in 11 days in 1962. A similar task was completed in 72 hours in 1969 and within one day in 1970. By the 1980s, new primary care teams were introduced, with a family practitioner and a nurse in every neighbourhood, covering just 600–700 people. (Waitzkin 1991: 171).

Professionals and patients

Investigating the relationships between medical professionals and their patients in Cuba, Howard Waitzkin, an American sociologist and physician, observes considerable contrasts with typical Western experience. This can be illustrated with one example, describing experiences encountered by one doctor.

While conducting her round the doctor came across an eleven-year-old boy who was experiencing problems at school, having detrimental consequences for his academic performance. The view of the boy's teachers was the he was 'mentally disturbed'. When school was finished the boy rarely left his house and preferred the company of his seventy-year-old grandmother, who was very protective. Waitzkin explains:

> On investigating further, the doctor learned that the boy was upset about a recent divorce of his parents. His father retained little contact with him, and his mother carried out extensive work responsibilities as a laboratory technician at a local hospital, where she often needed to work evening and night shifts. The grandmother suffered from anxiety, loneliness and osteoarthritis of the hands and feet that limited her activity, as well as hypertension controlled adequately with two medications.

The doctor proceeded to set up various meetings: with the boy's teachers, the coordinator of the neighbourhood's youth centre, a representative of People's Power, and the leaders of the 'grandparents' circle':

> Teenagers active at the youth centre visited the boy at home and asked him to get involved in the centre's activities, including the construction of a new wing of the building. He responded positively and enjoyed learning construction skills. His school work began to improve ...
>
> For other family members, the doctor also took action to improve the social situation. She discussed the mother's work schedule both with her and her superiors at the hospital, but changes had not yet proven possible. For the grandmother, leaders of the local grandparents' circle visited the home and

encouraged her participation in their activities. The grandmother then began to visit the grandparents' circle facility every day, where she socialized, watched television, and took part in a medically supervised exercise programme.

(Waitzkin 1991: 270)

Waitzkin goes on to report positive results from these interventions, but the example raises several important issues. At the core of these is the question of whether, by treating the patient as a person and responding to a wider range of factors than the immediate symptoms, health professionals enter areas of a person's life where they have no business.

Clinical consultations and social problems

For Western health care systems, Waitzkin advocates change in four key areas. First, participants in medical encounters should 'try to overcome the domination, mystification and distorted communication that result from asymmetric technical knowledge'. Second, 'doctors and patients should avoid the medicalization of non-medical problems' (Waitzkin 1991: 275–6).

These each relate to themes discussed in earlier chapters and it is perhaps in Waitzkin's third and fourth proposals that his more original approach lies. The third relates to a need to 'analyze the social origins of personal suffering', in which Waitzkin notes a doctor's participation may or may not be appropriate. However, he suggests several examples of circumstances where he believes the professional may be able to assist in identifying more relevant sources of support:

The health professional, for example, might refer a patient to a labour union, women's organization, cultural centre, community group, or other organization for assistance ... Organizations that aim towards outreach, advocacy, heightened democratic participation, and popular control should receive not only referrals but also other kinds of support from clinicians ... In the United States, several community-based programs already have tried to grapple in a systematic way with the contextual issues that affect patients; such efforts deserve every support.

(Waitzkin 1991)

Fourth, Waitzkin discusses the 'ideologic foundations of medical practice':

Physical illness may demand technical intervention as therapy, but social problems require resistance, activism and organizing ... When occupational toxins, stress of job insecurity produces symptoms, for instance, labor organizing is the preferred therapy, in addition to whatever physical treatment is appropriate. For the tension headaches and psychosomatic complaints of tedious housework, sexual politics aim directly at social causes. For alcoholism and other addictions that seek oblivion from the strains of social life, organizing at the level of local communities can begin to convert isolation to resistance. These rather facile examples oversimplify the clinical dilemma. The point, however, is that a progressive doctor–patient relationship fosters social change. Otherwise, the medical encounter dulls the pain of today, without hoping to extinguish it in the future.

(Waitzkin 1991: 276–7)

Many health professionals may feel that the solution to social problems experienced by patients lie well beyond their powers to control. Does this mean they have no role to play? Many practitioners might now regard it as appropriate to recommend that a patient contact an appropriate self-help group, but what about organizations dealing with social rather than clinical problems? Trade unions, community groups and other organizations might be better placed than many professionals to provide practical assistance for a range of problems.

Welfare benefit take-up by low-income patients

An example of the role non-clinical referral can play comes from projects designed to improve access to advice about welfare benefits. Research in this area is fairly limited but is beginning to point to the value of this type of advice, particularly when based within primary care. One study, based on a questionnaire sent to 153 inner city GPs, found a difference between the 81 that had specialist advisers in their surgery and the 72 that did not:

Those practitioners with specialist advisers in their surgery were significantly more likely to find referring patients to advisers easy, that quality of advice for patients was good, that welfare advisers enhanced their ability to practice effectively and that such provision improves the health and well-being of patients.

(Harding et al. 2003)

A smaller study looked in detail at the impact of providing welfare rights advice to a group of patients aged 65 and over who were judged by nurses to be physically or mentally frail. The setting was a general practice located on two sites in the East End of Glasgow, and 86 participants were identified by nurses, district nurses and health visitors. All were contacted by a welfare rights adviser, and 37 were found not to be receiving benefits to which they were entitled. Four relatives were also found to be in this position. For these 41 people, annually recurring benefits of nearly £100,000 were identified, in addition to £17,500 in non-recurring lump sums. The study concluded:

A community nurse-led attendance allowance screening service combined with a home visit by a Welfare Rights Officer was an efficient and highly effective model for maximizing the income of the frail elderly. This model could contribute to reducing the increasing number of pensioners living below the poverty line.

(Hoskins and Smith 2002)

An earlier review of literature on welfare rights advice in primary care settings suggests that this finding is typical (Hoskins and Carter 2000). For example, in the early 1990s, an Islington benefits project realized £300,000 in unclaimed benefit, from an initial investment of £20,000 and in two years the North Derbyshire 'Welfare Rights in Primary Care' project revealed an estimated unclaimed entitlement of £1,292,406, for an investment of £54,000.

Referring to an evaluation of a Liverpool-based project, Hoskins and Carter observe:

> although there were no statistically significant differences in primary care use before and after benefits advice, the general trend was for a decrease in consultations and prescriptions by those who received increased income and a corresponding increase by those who did not.
>
> (Hoskins and Carter 2000: 394)

They argue: 'Placing a welfare benefit uptake project in a primary care setting provides access to money advice to a whole range of vulnerable groups who would otherwise be excluded due to their age, poor health, poverty or lack of transport' (Hoskins and Carter 2000: 393).

Noting comments made by community nurses involved in a project in Wigan and Leigh, that they did not want to develop specialist welfare benefits knowledge but to know when it was appropriate to refer a client for this kind of advice, Hoskins and Carter conclude: 'If community nurses wish to make a major impact on improving the health of their clients they must not only promote healthy behaviour, but also attempt to improve disadvantaged life circumstances' (Hoskins and Carter 2000: 396).

Empowering or controlling the patient?

There are critics of developing professional practice in these directions. It may involve professionals in aspects of living that help determine ill-health, but to some this could epitomize the worst kind of 'nanny state'. This takes us back to the fundamental question about the responsibilities of individuals and the state.

Michael Fitzpatrick, in his book *The Tyranny of Health*, illustrates this in criticisms he levels at suggestions from Benzeval and Donald (1999: 94) that community-based health professionals can play a more active role in reducing health inequalities. One of their proposals was for more 'home visiting by health visitors, GPs and trained community peers to reinforce preventative health measures'.

Fitzpatrick rejects this approach: 'How could one conduct such a "reinforcement" visit? ... Under the banner of health inequalities, New Labour has turned health promotion into a sophisticated instrument for the regulation, not only of individual behaviour, but that of whole communities' (Fitzpatrick 1999).

Parallel arguments can be found in an article in which O'Brien (1994) claims that moving beyond narrow clinical categories may not produce the more patient-centred focus that is sometimes assumed. O'Brien explored nurses' approaches to dealing with health promotion, finding this tended to emphasize the importance of individual changes in behaviour. However, the article challenges the assumption that shifts towards a person-centred and 'holistic' model of care within nursing and other health professions should be seen in an entirely positive light. O'Brien argues that instead of being 'the ulcer in bed 5', the patient instead becomes 'the smoker from the estate' or 'the stressed manager'. In other words, classification by diagnostic category is replaced by one based on selected dimensions of behaviour. Wider influences on health were often neglected and: 'the ethics and politics of the control of information did not reach the agenda' (O'Brien 1994: 406).

Observing that the nurses employed emotional labour and interpersonal skills to alter clients' behaviour, O'Brien is concerned that this merely becomes an institutional resource to reinforce control over the health agenda by 'experts' and professionals.

The social context of personal control

This discussion introduces a further dimension to debates over the balance to be struck between the responsibilities of individuals and of the state. This concerns the factors that appear to be within the power of individuals to control and change, and those lying beyond.

In the nineteenth century there were those who argued that it was not the proper role of the state or its agents to introduce public water supply and sewerage systems. Typically these objections came from members of the middle class, who as ratepayers would be required to fund these developments. In the early years of urban growth, middle-class residential areas also tended to be largely spared the epidemics of infection that spread through the poorer sectors. This was to change but where the line is drawn between personal and public responsibility can have profound consequences for the social distribution of health.

In countries such as Britain, the character of illness has changed substantially since the infectious epidemics of the nineteenth century. This does not mean the environment in which we live is any less important but as physical environments improve, the influence of the social environment may grow.

Consider the following statistics, behind each of which lie personal stories, which together suggest trends that need to be explored and understood as social phenomena:

> Rates of suicide among males aged 15–24 rose from 6.9 per 1,000 to 16.4 per 1,000 between 1971 and 1997. Among 25–44 year old males the rate rose from 13.5 to 21.8, and by 2002 had risen to 24.1 per 1,000.
>
> (Social Trends 2000: 30; 2004: 34)
>
> In 1995, 25 per cent of men and 37 per cent of women aged 55–64 suffered back pain for a period of at least one month in the previous year.
>
> (Social Trends 2000: 30)
>
> Between 1994 and 1998, rates of treated depression among males living in prosperous areas were 22 per 1,000 and 57 per 1,000 for females. In deprived

industrial areas the rates were 34 per 1,000 for men and 77 per 1,000 for women.

(Social Trends 2001: 31)

The number of prescription items for anti-depressant drugs dispensed in England more than doubled between 1991 and 2001, from nine million to twenty four million.

(Social Trends 2003: 33)

Interpretation of these figures requires taking account of personal circumstances and social context. A generalized notion of 'the patient', as used in much of this book until now, is not always sufficient. It can help us explore general aspects of the patient experience, and interactions with professionals, but patients in reality differ not just as individuals but because of social characteristics. This may include the role of social class, gender, ethnicity, age and much else. The challenge of the sociological imagination is to appreciate consequences these have for the individual, without assuming stereotyped behaviour.

One important element of this relates to patterns of health and ill-health in society. Inequalities in health status between social groups are substantial, and in several areas are widening. This has particular significance in a context where opportunities for patient choice are receiving more and more emphasis. Will this, as the government predicts, result in a reduction of inequalities – or might the reverse occur? To introduce this debate and develop this focus, the next chapter considers key aspects of social inequalities in health.

7

The social distribution of health

A relationship between income and health has long been evident. Poorer people die younger, and have more illness, than their wealthier counterparts. Early interest in recording and measuring the social distribution of health, however, came not from epidemiologists or health specialists, but was stimulated by the need to calculate life insurance premiums.

The Society for Equitable Insurance on Lives and Survivorships was formed in 1762. An earlier attempt had been prevented by the Privy Council in the previous year, on the grounds that its proposed method for calculating risks of mortality was untested: 'the chance of mortality is attempted to be reduced to a certain standard: this is mere speculation, never yet tried in practice' (Cited in Stedman Jones 2004: 33).

Once the Society was established, premiums were calculated from bills of mortality in London, first by the mathematician James Dodson, and after his death, by another mathematician, and Welsh dissenting preacher, Richard Price. However, remarks by a Dr Hall, in 1805, suggest this had not allowed for differences in mortality between social groups:

> When the Equitable Insurance Office at Blackfriars Bridge was first established, the premiums taken were according to the ratio proposed by Dr Price, who formed it from the bills of mortality kept in different cities of Europe. These deaths were about 1 in 22, annually, of all the people, taken indiscriminately. Proceeding thus, the profits of the Society were so great, that in a few years they realised their enormous capital, upon which, their premiums were lowered ... The Society, not withstanding, continued to increase in riches. The cause of the phenomenon, therefore, was a matter of inquiry, on which it was found they had adapted their premiums to the deaths of the rich and poor together; and it soon occurred that none but the rich were insured. Their extraordinary profit, therefore, must arise from the circumstances of there being fewer deaths annually among the rich than among the poor, in proportion to the numbers of both ... it seems probable that the deaths of the poor are to those of the rich as two to one, in proportion to the numbers of each.
>
> (Cited in Davey Smith, Dorling, and Shaw 2001: xvii–xviii)

Health inequalities today

Remarkably, two centuries later, the ratio has changed little. At the very start of life, the infant mortality rate among children born to unskilled manual workers is about double that for children born to professional parents. Evidence of continuing disparities in health has prompted the government in recent years to give the issue much greater prominence, making use of statistics such as these taken from an official review:

> In Manchester, boys can expect to live almost eight years fewer, and girls almost seven years fewer than their contemporaries in Kensington, Chelsea and Westminster.
>
> Life expectancy for males in unskilled manual occupations is over seven years less than for professional social classes. For women the gap is over 5.5 years.
> (HM Treasury/Department of Health 2002: 1)

Greater attention on health inequalities by central government is resulting in growing pressure on local services to address the problem. Some aspects of this form the focus for a later chapter, on access to health services, but it is important to begin with a wider perspective. Without this, as an aid to improving the analysis of health inequalities, there are risks that policy intentions will not achieve the desired outcomes. This is alluded to in a study of midwifery services, in which the authors suggest that despite: 'a genuine commitment on the part of the current government to address health inequalities ... this is matched by vagueness within the documents about who those clients are, and what the practitioners should actually be doing in relation to them' (Hart and Lockey 2002: 486).

There is, though, a prior question to address even before ways of analysing health inequalities are considered. This concerns the justification for treating health inequalities as a matter of importance for policy and professional practice. It can be argued that, although there is evidence of continuing inequalities in health, this is to a large extent offset by the enormous improvements in health that have benefited all social groups. For example, in York in 1900 one child in four living in the poorest parts of the city died before reaching their first birthday, compared to one child in ten among the richest groups (Marmot 2004: 64–5). In Britain today, fewer than one in a hundred children born to the very poorest parents die in the first year of life.

Targets have, nevertheless, been set for the National Health Service to reduce inequalities in infant mortality. In the context of this huge improvement, are these really justified?

Do health inequalities matter?

A critic of several aspects of current health policy, the writer and GP Michael Fitzpatrick, makes the point: 'the government and the medical profession have become more preoccupied with the relationship between inequality and health at a time when social differentials in health are less significant in real terms than ever before' (Fitzpatrick 1999: 4).

Saying this, he does not ignore the evidence of inequalities. He refers to data showing that infant mortality among babies whose fathers are in unskilled manual occupations was 11.7 per 1000 live births in 1990, compared to 6.2 per 1000 among babies born to professional parents. However, he goes on: 'While there can be little doubt that the persistence of this differential is a pernicious effect of Britain's class divided society, it is important to place it in a wider context' (Fitzpatrick 1999: 4–5).

This wider context includes the substantial reductions in infant mortality achieved throughout the twentieth century. At the turn of the nineteenth/twentieth centuries the death rate was around 150 per 1000 live births, and by the time of the Second World War it was still above 50 per 1000. Not until the 1960s did the rate fall below 20 (Halsey 1988), but in 1990 the overall death rate was slightly less than eight per 1000 live births and by 1996 it had fallen below six. There were 3390 infant deaths in 1990, compared with 142,912 in 1900.

Fitzpatrick points out that infant mortality has fallen dramatically among all social classes in the course of the twentieth century. For example, in 1922 infant mortality among unskilled workers was 97 per 1000 and for professionals 38 per 1000 (Halsey 1988), and:

> Over the past 70 years, the rate has fallen to roughly the same extent – between 80 and 90 per cent – among both the richest and the poorest. The infant mortality rate among the poorest families today is similar to that of the richest in the 1970s.
>
> Though infant deaths may be relatively more common in poorer families, they are very uncommon in any section of society ... Furthermore, many of these deaths result from conditions such as prematurity and congenital abnormalities, which are often difficult to prevent, or are 'cot deaths', the causes of which are uncertain and preventive measures remain controversial. Again, it seems that the level of government and official medical intervention is out of all proportion to the scale of the problem.
>
> (Fitzpatrick 1999: 5)

A similar viewpoint has been advanced in an analysis published in *The Lancet* of a report by the London Health Observatory. The original report compared infant mortality rates between London boroughs, which showed: 'Bexley was the borough that had the lowest infant mortality rate of 3.6 infant deaths per 1000 live births and Hackney was the borough which had the highest infant mortality rate of 8.9 infant deaths per 1000 live births' (Oliver *et al.* 2002).

However, the writers argue:

> if we translate these figures into raw probabilities, we show that the chance of an infant dying if born in Hackney is around 0.005 higher than if that same infant were born in Bexley. If we want to increase societal welfare, we have to

reason whether this 0.005 difference in absolute probability of infant mortality represents a substantial inequity, and whether it is worthy of the possible substantial resource injections that would be needed to reduce it.

(Oliver *et al.* 2002)

Another example used in *The Lancet* article is drawn from a comparison of mortality rates in the US, which suggested these were 'nearly twice as high for individuals with incomes under $7500 than for those making more than $32,500 a year'. However, Oliver *et al.* point out that when the respective rates are expressed as probabilities, the average probability for the two groups is 0.004 and 0.008:

Before we assume that this 0.004 difference in the probability of death is an inequity that should be addressed, we have to provide a clear rationale for why it is an inequity, and if so, whether investment in policy interventions to reduce it would represent best use of scarce societal resources.

In our view, it is important that governments around the world do not get too embroiled with the views of people who treat alleviation of health inequalities as an agenda to be addressed without due consideration of other health-related policy objectives. A substantial reduction in health inequality in any country will probably entail considerable resources, great opportunity costs, and an extensive timeframe.

(Oliver *et al.* 2002: 566)

The arguments advanced by Fitzpatrick and Oliver *et al.* are similar. Basically they are saying that although the ratio of deaths between poorer and richer groups in society has remained much the same over the past century, the scale of reduction in both groups has been enormous. This means that the actual numbers of excess deaths among poorer groups is now very small. No one is questioning the significance of these for the families involved, but the question is put about whether investing substantial resources to seek further reductions is justified. For a utilitarian calculation, does this represent the most effective use of resources?

Inequalities, risk and probability

Before tackling this directly, it is worth pausing to comment on the concept of probability: the likelihood or chance of something happening. When we say there is a 'fifty-fifty' chance of an event occurring, we are indicating a probability. It could just as well be stated as a percentage; in this case it would be 50 per cent. Probabilities are more frequently expressed as proportions, so that if something does not happen, or there is no chance of it occurring, there is a probability of 0. Likewise, if something happens or is certain to happen, there is a probability of 1. If I toss a coin there is a 50 per cent chance of it landing heads and a 50 per cent chance of it being tails. Each can be expressed as a probability of 0.5. The sum of the probabilities of all possible outcomes will always be 1.

Probability ratios are a valuable tool for making comparisons between events but because the sum total of all possible outcomes will always be 1, differences in probabilities between alternative results can appear quite small. This can be illustrated with a different health-related example.

Department of Health data on cases of reported food poisoning show that in 1990 there were 49,122 known cases of food poisoning in England, a figure that had risen to 81,812 by 2000. Now if we express these as probabilities, with a population in England of slightly over 49 million (2001 census), we find that the probability of contracting food poisoning in 1990 was about 0.0010 and in 2000 was 0.0017. The difference in probability is 0.0007 but both are very low.

Nevertheless, this represents nearly 82,000 people who probably became quite ill in the course of a single year because of food poisoning, a two-thirds increase over a ten-year period. The increased probability of 0.0007 represents about 32,000 people.

Returning to the example of infant mortality rates across London boroughs, it is undoubtedly true that the probability of infant mortality in both Hackney and Bexley is very low. However, making comparisons across large time periods is not always relevant for interpreting contemporary inequalities. Infant mortality rates of today and those of 1900 are separated by a century of social, nutritional and medical advances. Between Bexley and Hackney there is no more than ten miles. The numbers of children who die in a single London borough is thankfully small but cumulatively, as all poorer areas are compared to more affluent ones, the numbers rise:

> If all infants and children up to age 15 enjoyed the same survival chances as the children from classes I and II (professional and intermediate occupations), then over 3,000 deaths a year might be prevented. Bringing all adults aged 16–64 up to the mortality experience of class I (professional) would mean 39,000 fewer deaths.
>
> (Whitehead 1992: 229)

This equates to about 115 deaths every single day of the year. Over a period of just ten years it would represent around 425,000 deaths; equivalent to the population of a city the size of Bristol. If deaths on this scale occurred in contexts such as rail transport or air flight, urgent action would be demanded by politicians and the public. Expressing the risks as a probability would do little to reassure. Problems need also to be defined on a more human scale.

This also requires us to look beyond the mortality data: the tip of a much larger iceberg of illness and incapacity. Blaxter makes the point that much of the debate on health inequalities has focused on mortality data:

> However, the general increase in life expectancy (principally due to the control of fatal communicable diseases and the reduction of infant deaths) has meant mortality rates which are generally low, before old age, and this not always clearly discriminatory. Inequalities in health may not be the same as inequalities in death.
>
> (Blaxter 1990: 7)

The scale of these inequalities in health, rather than in mortality, can be illustrated by using data from the 2001 census on self-reported, limiting long-term illness. This is summarized in the map below, indicating the proportion of people in each local authority area who reported having a limiting long-term illness.

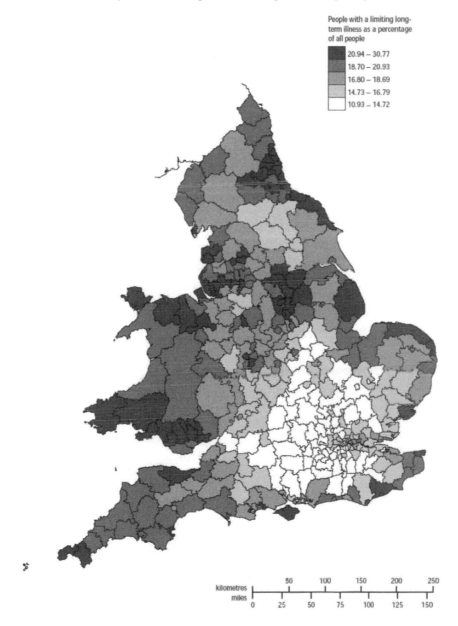

Figure 7.1 Limiting long-term illness

A further reason for seeing health inequalities as a problem requiring attention is that they appear not only to be persisting, but are widening. Between 1972 and 1996, men in professional occupations experienced a rise in life expectancy of 5.7 years: the increase was of just 1.7 years for unskilled manual workers (Hattersley 1999). This has meant that the death rate among professionals has gone from being double that for unskilled manual workers in the 1970s, to a threefold difference by the 1990s (Graham 2000: 9). This is associated with very important differences between geographical localities and, as one study has concluded: 'geographical inequalities in mortality now stand at the highest levels ever recorded' (Dorling, Shaw and Brimblecombe 2000).

On these three grounds – that the number of excess deaths among poorer groups remains high despite considerable improvements; that inequalities in mortality reflect a far larger number of people experiencing pain and incapacity; and that indicators show inequalities are widening rather than narrowing – I am unconvinced by claims that excessive attention is being directed towards the problem of health inequalities.

Responding to health inequalities

How inequalities should be tackled presents a more complex problem. This question has caused governments of different political affiliations to hesitate in confronting the issues head-on. In the early 1980s, the then Conservative Government's Secretary of State for Health, Patrick Jenkin, refused to endorse the recommendations of a committee established to investigate inequalities in health, on the grounds that the spending required was prohibitive:

> the Group has reached the view that the causes of health inequalities are so deep-rooted that only a major and wide-ranging programme of public expenditure is capable of altering the pattern. I must make it clear that additional expenditure on the scale which could result from the report's recommendations – the amount involved could be upwards of £2 billion a year – is quite unrealistic in present or any foreseeable economic circumstances, quite apart from any judgement that may be formed of the effectiveness of such expenditure in dealing with the problems identified. I cannot, therefore, endorse the Group's recommendations. I am making the report available for discussion, but without any commitment by the government to its proposals.
>
> (Townsend and Davidson 1982: 39)

Current government policy shows greater readiness to recognize the importance of health inequalities but this is still accompanied by a guarded approach towards public expenditure. Concerns about making substantial investment in this area of policy may not result from a failure to consider the issue an important one, but reflect Patrick Jenkin's question about the 'effectiveness of expenditure'. What is the point of spending large amounts of public money if the precise causes and origins of health inequalities are inadequately understood? On this issue debate still rages; with conflicting views supported by competing evidence. This chapter does not attempt a thorough review of these debates but seeks to chart a passage through them.

Many ways of categorizing different approaches to explaining health inequalities exist but a reasonably simple, threefold distinction distinguishes material, behavioural and psychosocial factors (Graham 2000). Although it is recognized that many health influences fall between and across these categories, they can be considered separately:

> Material factors include the physical environment of the home, neighbour-hood and workplace, together with living standards secured through earnings, benefits and other income. Behavioural factors are the health-related routines and habits which display a strong socio-economic gradient, like cigarette smoking, leisure-time exercise and diet...
>
> Alongside of the material and behavioural determinants, research is uncover-ing the psychosocial costs of living in an unequal society. For example, perceiving oneself to be worse off relative to others may carry a health penalty, in terms of increased stress and risk-taking behaviour.
>
> (Graham 2000: 14–15)

This chapter, and the two that follow, will be largely organized around these themes. In this chapter, issues relating to both material and behavioural factors will be considered, beginning with a short historical account of the association between poverty and ill-health. 'Psychosocial' factors provide the focus for the next two chapters. Reasons for this structure and balance are twofold. First, and straight-forwardly, it is in the area of psychosocial origins of illness that some of the more recent research and debate has arisen. Summaries of it are, therefore, less readily accessible than is the case for longer-standing debates about the role of poverty and individual behaviour.

The re-emergence of psychosocial explanations

The second reason requires a little more explanation. The term 'psychosocial' was introduced in the previous chapter in relation to Halliday's advocacy of 'psycho-social medicine'. Ways in which it has come to be used more recently are explained in an account of the 'psychosocial perspective':

> The term 'perspective' is chosen because I consider it a set of related approaches rather than a unified theory. It can, however, be identified by three core assumptions: (1) the distribution of psychological stress is an important determinant of health inequalities in present-day affluent societies, (2) psy-chological stress is strongly influenced by the quality of social and inter-personal relations, and (3) the latter are determined to a large extent by the magnitude of society's inequalities.
>
> (Elstad 1998: 40)

A shorter, and even broader definition has been provided by Marmot (2004: 123), who describes psychosocial factors as being 'psychological factors that are influenced by the social environment'. As is hopefully evident by now, this essentially describes much of the approach adopted in this book, seeking to link individual biographical experiences with wider societal influences.

A problem is that such all-encompassing definitions open up a potentially enormous field of enquiry. However valid it is to emphasize the impact of 'domestic, economic and political society' upon an individual and their health, the umbrella term of 'psychosocial factors' does little to specify the particular routes that may be involved. 'Psychosocial' provides a useful portmanteau word, indicating the importance of interaction between the social and the personal, but at a level of generality that is insufficient to guide us in exploring specific channels of transmission.

Most writers in this area have identified what they consider to be the primary routes through which psychosocial factors operate. For example, Richard Wilkinson gives particular emphasis to the role of income inequalities, noting that the notion of relative income is an inherently social concept: 'It reflects an aspect of the relationship of an individual to a social group' (Wilkinson 1996: 175).

Wilkinson argues that more unequal societies are more fragmented with, he suggests, lower levels of 'social capital', a notion that: 'refers to connections among individuals – social networks and the norms of reciprocity and trustworthiness that arise from them' (Putnam 2000: 19).

Wilkinson does not deny the damaging effect on health of living in poor material circumstances. The health consequences of bad housing, for example, are well attested. However, he suggests that in a country such as Britain, an absolute lack of material resources cannot explain the continuing prevalence of inequalities. Suggesting instead that 'we need to put together a combination of what is summed up by the notions of social cohesion and civilization' (Wilkinson 1996: 220), he identifies the specific role of:

> social affiliations and social support, a sense of control and of security. In addition, social cohesion relates easily to the sense of coherence which Antonovsky and others have suggested is protective of health . . . If there is not a sense of social justice, then the legitimacy of social institutions is fundamentally weakened and the moral community which makes social life coherent is lacking. Cohesion and coherence are therefore likely to closely relate to social justice.
>
> (Wilkinson 1996: 220–1)

These are important and intriguing suggestions but there is a need for clarity about the particular process involved. This is attempted in the subsequent two chapters, which utilize long-standing concepts within sociology to establish a framework for thinking about different forms that psychosocial factors may take.

Social relationships and work and control

Beginning with the social relationships in which we lead our everyday lives (friends, families and communities), attention is given to their importance as sources of social support, and evidence is provided on the relationship between social support and health status. This develops to consider the wider argument made in relation to social capital, that social networks of this kind are important building blocks for good health.

Related to the character of social networks in society are the social values and norms through which individuals feel a sense of belonging. This provides an opportunity to introduce the concept of anomie, which describes situations in which the norms governing social interaction break down. Associated with the French sociologist, Emil Durkheim, the concept is based on the idea that human behaviour requires social regulation to restrain individuals from acting excessively. A state of anomie occurs where this is absent. However, for Durkheim, rules alone were not enough to prevent this: 'The mere existence of rules is not sufficient: they must also be just' (Durkheim 1997: 338).

Referring to social disruption of a century ago, he rejected ideas that former traditions and practices could be revived but argued:

> We need to put a stop to this anomie, and to find ways of harmonious co-operation between those organs that still clash discordantly together. We need to introduce into their relationships a greater justice by diminishing those external inequalities that are the source of our ills.
>
> (p. 340)

Durkheim's attention to inequality as a source of anomie provides an opportunity to consider some of Richard Wilkinson's work. I have chosen to differentiate this from discussion on community and social capital because there are important differences. While the notion of social capital relates to how far we feel socially integrated, the concept of anomie refers to the extent to which we allow our behaviour to be regulated by society. Both form an important focus for Chapter 8.

In Chapter 9, attention turns to what Wilkinson in the extract above refers to as 'control and security'. This is an aspect to which Michael Marmot draws particular attention: 'autonomy – how much control you have over your life – and the opportunities you have for full social engagement and participation are crucial for health, well-being and longevity' (Marmot 2004: 2).

In giving attention to issues of control in the workplace, the discussion in Chapter 9 draws on the work of the German political philosopher, Karl Marx, and in particular, his interest in changing experiences of work and the concept of alienation.

The remainder of this chapter focuses on the role of material and behavioural factors. In the middle of the nineteenth century, writers as diverse as Frederick Engels, Karl Marx's lifelong collaborator, and the civil servant Edwin Chadwick, chronicled examples of appalling standards of health. Most wretched were some of the poorest parts of the newly industrializing towns and cities. In his 1844 account, *The Condition of the Working Class in England,* Engels observes:

> Typhus, that universally diffused affliction, is attributed by the official report on the sanitary condition of the working class, directly to the bad state of the dwellings in the matters of ventilation, drainage and cleanliness ... But the fury of the epidemic in all former periods seems to have been child's play in comparison with its ravages after the crisis of 1842. One-sixth of the whole indigent population of Scotland was seized by the fever, and the infection was carried by wandering beggars with fearful rapidity from one locality to another. It did not reach the middle and upper classes of the population, yet in two months there were more fever cases than in twelve years before. In Glasgow twelve per cent of the population were seized in the year 1843; 32,000 persons, of whom thirty two per cent perished...
>
> (Engels 1969: 129–31)

For Engels, and his contemporaries, the terms 'working class' and 'poor' were virtually synonymous. In subsequent years, the relationship between the two has altered, with changes in the experiences of different sections of the working population. For this reason, it is appropriate to consider the relationship between health and class, and health and poverty separately, beginning with the concept of social class.

Social class and health

Many commentators, politicians and social scientists believe social class to be of declining importance in contemporary society. This is not necessarily because social inequalities are assumed to be a thing of the past. Ulrich Beck, for example, gives great emphasis to the fact that these are widening (Beck 1992). At issue is the relevance of the *concept* of class for understanding social experiences and identities. Is it a category that resonates with people's own sense of who they are?

Class, as a form of social identity, is not the only way in which the term can be used. It also provides a basis of social classification that is frequently used in comparisons of health status between different groups in society. This involves using the category of class as a way of placing individuals within a pre-defined classification system, which may bear little relation to how those individuals would perceive and describe their own class position.

The historian, E.P. Thompson, had little patience with sociological definitions of class that were not grounded in people's own sense of identity:

> By class I understand a historical phenomenon, unifying a number of disparate and seemingly unconnected events, both in the raw material of experience and in consciousness. I do not see class as a 'structure', nor even as a 'category', but as something which in fact happens (and can be shown to have happened) in human relationships ...

The finest-meshed sociological net cannot give us a pure specimen of class, any more than it can give us one of deference or of love. The relationship must always be embodied in real people and a real context...

Class is defined by men as they live their own history, and, in the end, this is its only definition.

(Thompson 1980: 8–10)

Such pleas to consider subjective meaning have not dissuaded many social scientists from trying to construct classificatory frameworks. Differences between approaches have been considerable but two deserve mention here because of their frequent use in comparisons of health and mortality data.

Registrar General's scale

One of the longest-standing occupational class schemes is the Registrar General's scale. Although it has been replaced recently in official statistics, much published analysis of social inequalities in health make use of it. The aim of the Registrar General's classification is to arrive at reasonably homogenous groupings of occupations, within a hierarchy determined by the occupations' 'general standing within the community'. Thus it is a measure of social status, not income or wealth (although there may be a relationship between status and these factors). Occupational categories underwent amendment during the years after 1913, when it was first introduced, and recent data is likely to be shown in a form that uses the following:

Table 7.1 Occupational categories

	Categories	Examples
I	Professional	Accountant, doctor, lawyer
II	Managerial and technical intermediate	Sales manager, teacher, journalist, nurse
IIIN	Skilled non-manual	Secretary, shop assistant, cashier
IIIM	Skilled manual	Joiner, bus driver, cook
IV	Semi-skilled manual worker	Security guard, machine tool operator, farm worker
V	Unskilled manual	Building labourer, cleaner, laundry worker

(From Graham 2000: 5)

Despite its wide use over many years, several problems are associated with this classification. Many arise from the fact that, although amended, the basic structure of the schema originated in the early years of the twentieth century. At that time the meaning of 'professional work', for instance, was very different to that half a century later, by which time the expansion of health, education and other public services had brought large changes to the composition of the workforce. Many of the new public sector professional groups did not enjoy the kind of social prestige that a professional might have expected before World War I and so were classified as 'intermediate' occupations. Another source of difficulty was the growth in managerial occupations, many of which did not fit easily into the schema as whole.

Problems arising from changes in the character of the labour force reflect a more fundamental issue. This derives from the basis on which ranking is done; in the Registrar General's schema the key criterion is perceived social prestige or status. The significance of this is illustrated in comments made by T.H.C. Stevenson, a medical statistician who originated the scale, in an article published in 1928:

> The power of culture to exert a favourable influence upon mortality, even in the complete absence of wealth, is well illustrated in the case of clergy. Their mortality is remarkably low. Of 178 occupation groups dealt with in the recently-published report on occupational mortality in 1921–23, Anglican clergy occupied second place.
> (Quoted in Davey-Smith, Dorling and Shaw 2001: 162)

Stevenson is very clear that social status provided the basis for differentiating between occupations. From this perspective, nothing about the occupation itself is assumed to correlate with health status. The importance of occupation derives from its perceived source of social prestige, rather than any inherent features. This emphasis is an important one because it distinguishes scales such as the Registrar General's from others that focus primarily on characteristics of occupations themselves.

In a discussion on the distinction between class and status, although in some contexts the concepts are used interchangeably, Rosemary Crompton suggests that, 'whereas "class" is concerned with the production of goods, status is concerned with their consumption' (Crompton 1993: 129). This may include a wide range of lifestyle features, manner of dress, speech, diet and much else. These are difficult to measure in any simple way, which is why the use of occupation as a proxy can appear attractive. But as occupations and social attitudes change, the relevance of previous categories inevitably diminishes. One of the problems with the Registrar General's scale was that the use of occupation gave the appearance that it was defining class by location within the workforce, whereas it was the assumed status that went with this that was really the focus. This created difficulties for interpreting the inequalities in health that the scale reveals. How are these to be explained? Which are the aspects of the occupational classification that are judged important?

National Statistics Socio-Economic Classification

Statisticians and social scientists responded to these problems by creating an alternative system of classification, the National Statistics Socio-Economic Classification (NS-SEC). From 2001, this has been used in official statistics, replacing the Registrar General's scale. The conceptual basis of the classification lies in the character of employment relations:

The NS-SEC aims to differentiate positions within labour markets and production units in terms of their typical 'employment relations'. Among
employees, there are quite diverse employment relations and conditions, that
is, they occupy different labour market situations and work situations. Labour
market situation equates to source of income, economic security and prospects
of economic advancement. Work situation refers primarily to location in
systems of authority and control at work, although degree of autonomy at work
is a secondary aspect. The NS-SEC categories thus distinguish different
positions as defined by social relationships in the workplace – i.e. by how
employees are regulated by employers through employment contracts. Three
forms of employment regulation are distinguished:

1. In a 'service relationship' the employee renders 'service' to the employer in
    return for 'compensation', in terms of both immediate rewards (e.g. sal-
    ary) and long-term or prospective benefits (e.g. assurances of security and
    career opportunities).
2. In a 'labour contract' employees give discrete amounts of labour in return
    for a wage calculated on amount of work done or by time worked.
3. Intermediate forms of employment regulation that combine aspects from
    both forms (1) and (2).

(Office for National Statistics 2004: 3–4)

The system is based upon eight categories:

1. Higher managerial and professional occupations
2. Lower managerial and professional occupations
3. Intermediate occupations
4. Small employers and own account workers
5. Lower supervisory and technical occupations
6. Semi-routine occupations
7. Routine occupations
8. Never worked and long-term unemployed

The first categories in this list would be regarded as service relationships, while
lower supervisory, technical, semi-routine and routine occupations would typify a
labour contract relationship. By basing categories on what are judged to be
important differences in experiences of work and employment, the classification
system aims to facilitate better explanations for statistical associations:

As the NS-SEC is measuring employment relations, i.e. aspects of work and
market situations and of the labour contract, the user can more readily construct causal narratives that specify how the NS-SEC links to a range of
outcomes via a variety of intervening variables.

(p. 3)

The rationale for this classificatory system is that it is based on explicit characteristics of jobs, in terms of the employment relationship in which they are performed, including factors such as security, authority and control. This, it is claimed, provides a stronger basis for explaining an association with indicators such as those of health status, than is possible with a more subjective, status-based schema such as the Registrar General's. To illustrate the two systems, the following two tables show examples of health data, using the Registrar General's schema and the NS-SEC.

Table 7.2 Distribution of coronary heart disease deaths by social class, using the Registrar General's occupational class schema (men aged 20–64) (1999)

Social class	Share of population (%)	Share of CHD deaths (%)	Number of CHD deaths (1999)
I	8	5	523
II	29	20	2249
IIIn	11	11	1268
IIIm	32	38	4295
IV	15	18	2007
V	5	9	1078

Source: HM Treasury/Department of Health 2004. Annex C: Figure 15

Table 7.3 Summary of responses to GHS (2001) questions on health by socio-economic category (Great Britain, males)

	Chronic sickness	Acute sickness	GP consultation
Large employers and higher managerial	13%	12%	10%
Higher professional	12%	11%	10%
Lower managerial and professional	15%	11%	9%
Intermediate	16%	9%	10%
Small employers and own account	17%	12%	11%
Lower supervisory and technical	21%	15%	13%
Semi-routine	21%	13%	12%
Routine	27%	17%	15%
Long-term unemployed	22%	17%	14%

Source: General Household Survey (2001)

Both sets of data show clear and substantial gradients declining from the higher to the lower occupational categories. Because the conceptual basis of the two classification systems are considerably different, caution is needed before making inferences about the causal factors that may be involved. The two tables indicate that health status appears to correlate both with a measure based on social status, and with one based on employment relationships. How is this to be inter-preted? What are the precise factors that might be involved?

These questions have generated considerable research and debate, and one approach to reviewing this is to draw a distinction between approaches in terms of the emphasis they give to material factors, such as income, and behavioural ones, particularly lifestyles.

Income, poverty and health

In 1899, Seebohm Rowntree, a Quaker and a director of the chocolate factory in York, sponsored a survey intended to identify the extent of poverty in the city. He used the term 'primary poverty' to describe circumstances in which the total earnings of families were 'insufficient to obtain the minimum necessaries for the maintenance of merely physical efficiency'. The maintenance of physical efficiency was regarded as requiring basic essentials, including food, clothing, housing and heating. Drawing on the work of nutritionists, Rowntree estimated adult and child nutritional needs, going on to calculate what food would be necessary to supply these and the cost. Adding other costs, representing essentials such as clothing and fuel, Rowntree arrived at a figure below which a family was deemed to be in 'primary poverty'. The figure was adjusted to take account of differing family size, being for example, 17s 8d a week for a couple with three children. Rowntree expressed the view:

> My poverty line represented the minimum sum on which physical efficiency could be maintained. It was a standard of bare *subsistence* rather than *living*. The diet I selected was more economical and less attractive than was given to paupers in workhouses. I purposely selected such a diet so that no one could possibly accuse me of placing my subsistence level too high.
>
> (Rowntree 1941)

Rowntree's desire was to establish an objective, measurable definition of poverty, but it has met criticism. Townsend (1974) points out that despite the intended objectivity, Rowntree's estimates of cost for non-food items were based on his own or others' opinions, or actual expenditure by a small sample of poor families. Does this tell us what really needs to be spent? Even for food, where nutritional evidence was used, estimates were averages, with little account taken of factors such as age, activity and occupation. Foods selected as a means of pro-viding the basic nutritional needs tended to be the cheapest available, rather than those most likely to be eaten. When compared with actual family expenditure, Rowntree's estimate of what spending was needed on food tended to be con-siderably higher (Townsend 1974: 17).

These problems illustrate some of the inherent difficulties in establishing an objective measure of poverty. To use a contemporary definition, the United Nations has defined 'absolute poverty' as: 'a condition characterised by severe deprivation of basic human needs, including food, safe drinking water, sanitation facilities, health, shelter, education and information' (United Nations 1995: 57).

On this definition, poverty would have been widespread in parts of Britain in the mid-nineteenth century but far more limited today. Globally, poverty on this scale remains an enormous cause of human suffering. According to the World Food Programme, the world's largest international aid agency, 25,000 people die of hunger and associated disease every day. That is equivalent to one death every four seconds. Seventy per cent of these are children (Arie and Burke 2004: 18).

Can the same word, poverty, really be used to describe deprivation, far less extreme but nonetheless capable of having a considerable impact on lifetime experiences and opportunities? Many writers believe it can.

The concept of relative poverty

One early example is the political economist Adam Smith, who suggested that poverty was the absence of: 'not only the commodities which are indispensably necessary for the support of life, but whatever the custom of the country renders it indecent for creditable people, even of the lowest order, to be without' (Smith 1804).

Writing in the mid-1960s, Brian Abel-Smith and Peter Townsend make a similar point about the definition of the word poverty: 'In any objective sense the word has no absolute meaning which can be applied in all societies at all times. Poverty is a relative concept. Saying who is in poverty is to make a relative statement – rather like saying who is short or heavy' (Abel-Smith and Townsend 1965: 63).

In later work, Peter Townsend went on to argue that poverty needed to be defined as a form of relative deprivation. This is a concept examined by Runciman (1972), who describes it as being first used in a large social-psychological study by Samuel Stouffer, conducted within the US army during the Second World War. The notion is a straightforward one: describing a situation where one person wants something that another has, and regards possession of it as feasible (Runciman 1972).

Drawing upon this concept, Townsend argues:

> Poverty can be described objectively and applied consistently only in terms of the concept of relative deprivation ... The term is understood objectively rather than subjectively. Individuals, families and groups in the population can be said to be in poverty when they lack the resources to obtain the types of diets, participate in the activities and have the living conditions and amenities which are customary, or are at least widely encouraged or approved, in the societies to which they belong.
>
> (Townsend 1974: 15)

This view was shared by the 1980 Black Report into inequalities in health, to which Townsend was a contributor:

> Poverty is also a relative concept, and those who are unable to share the amenities or facilities provided within a rich society, or who are unable to fulfil

the social and occupational obligations placed upon them by virtue of their limited resources, can properly be regarded as poor. They may also be relatively disadvantaged in relation to the risks of illness or accident or the factors positively promoting health.

(Townsend and Davidson 1982: 115)

Using this approach, Townsend constructed a list of sixty indicators of 'style of living'. The list included: 'diet, clothing, fuel and light, home amenities and housing facilities, the immediate environment of the home, the characteristics, security, general conditions and welfare benefits at work, family support, recreation, education, health and social relations' (Townsend 1979: 249–51).

The list was incorporated into a questionnaire, used to explore the relationship between styles of living and household income. Questions asked included ones such as, whether a holiday away from home had been taken in the previous 12 months, or an evening out in the preceding two weeks, as well as others about the possession of household equipment, such as refrigerators, and type of meals (Townsend 1979: 250). Looking at the list today is a reminder of how much has changed since the 1970s but this illustrates Townsend's main claim: that definitions of poverty must relate to a particular social context.

Poverty or inequality?

Subsequent work, by Townsend and others, has explored the relationship between indices of deprivation and health status, demonstrating that the association is a very close one. Almost everywhere, as deprivation increases, so too does the prevalence of poor health. This might suggest that a lack of material resources, and the consequences this has for style of living, are to be seen as among the most important determinants. However, it is necessary to remember that the approach is one that is based upon a relative concept of poverty. The material standard of living associated with it will change with prevailing social conditions and expectations. For this reason, Townsend's approach to defining poverty has been criticized. David Piachaud, for example, has argued:

Social scientists can describe the inequality of resources within and between countries as objectively as possible. *But inequality is not the same as poverty.* The term 'poverty' carries with it an implication and moral imperative that something should be done about it. The definition by an individual, or by a society collectively, of what level represents 'poverty', will always be a value-judgement. Social scientists have no business trying to pre-empt such judgements with 'scientific' prescriptions.

(Piachaud 1993: 119)

This debate is one that cannot be adequately explored here, but it brings to the fore the consequences of defining poverty in an absolute or relative manner. Arguments for taking the latter course are compelling but if this is done is it not, as Piachaud suggests, inequality that really becomes the focus? And if this is so, why should inequality – rather than inadequate material resources – affect health status? This question runs through much of the work by Richard Wilkinson.

The social distribution of health

Using a large amount of data from different countries, Wilkinson seeks to explain what has been described as the 'epidemiological transition':

> The term is used to demarcate the change from predominantly infectious causes of death, still common in poor countries, to the degenerative diseases which have become the predominant cause of death in richer countries...
>
> The epidemiological transition seems to mark a more fundamental turning point in history than is usually recognised. As well as the decline in infections, it also marks a change in the social distribution of a number of important conditions. During the 'epidemiological transition' the so-called 'diseases of affluence' became the diseases of the poor in affluent countries. The most well-known example is coronary heart disease which, in the first half of the twentieth century, was regarded as a businessman's disease but changed its social distribution to become more common in lower social classes. Several other causes of death, including stroke, hypertension, duodenal ulcers, nephritis and nephrosis, and suicide also reversed their social distribution to become more common among the least well-off.
>
> (Wilkinson 1996: 43–4)

Obesity provides a particularly important example. Once it had been the rich who were fatter, while the poor were thin, causing obesity to be regarded as a desirable status symbol through much of human history. Wilkinson's point is that although material resources matter a great deal for health up to a certain point, beyond this threshold they no longer exert any significant influence. Since the 1950s, for instance, the proportion of babies born in Britain weighing less than 2500 grams has remained around 6–7 per cent, despite substantial rises in real incomes since then. This, argues Wilkinson 'suggests that the remaining part of the problem of low birthweights is unlikely to be directly attributable to absolute material living standards' (Wilkinson 1996: 45).

With only a very small proportion of the population in developed societies living with basic material deprivation, it is to the effects of 'relative deprivation' that Wilkinson turns his attention (Wilkinson 1996: 46). The result of his analysis of various sources of international comparative data is the conclusion:

> Countries in which the income differences between the rich and poor are larger (meaning more or deeper relative poverty) tend to have worse health than countries in which the differences are smaller. It is ... the most egalitarian rather than the richest developed countries which have the best health.
>
> (Wilkinson 1996: 75)

Wilkinson's work has not been without its critics, and others have argued that the results can depend upon which particular countries are included in the comparison (see, for example, Judge 1995). Some of these debates take the form of technical methodological disputes, which cannot be pursued here. There is, though, a more fundamental question. Even if a correlation of the kind suggested does exist, this does not in itself provide evidence of a causal relationship. Evidence of a different kind would be needed to establish this case firmly, but the nature of the problem makes this extremely difficult to identify.

One possibility might be to move below the comparisons between countries, to examine inequalities within countries. We know that the scale of inequalities in health varies between regions, with London and Scotland showing the greatest disparities. Among men in both areas about 35 per 1000 of those in higher managerial and professional occupations described their health as 'not good', compared to approximately 100 per 1000 in routine occupations and 200 per 1000 among those who were long-term unemployed or who had never worked (Doran, Drever and Whitehead 2004). If the argument that inequalities in health are associated with wider inequalities is valid, it might be expected that those regions with the greatest health inequalities would also show the widest inequalities in wealth.

Evidence to support this is limited. One relevant study sought to test the hypothesis that 'people in regions of Britain with the greatest income inequality would report worse health than those in other regions'. The results indicated that higher scores on one particular measure of inequality, the Gini index, were associated with worse self-rated health, particularly among those on the lowest incomes. However, other measures of inequality did not show this same relationship. Aside from these issues about measurement, it was also noted that regions with the highest inequalities in income were also those with the largest urban populations, raising the possibility that this – rather than inequalities – might be the determining factor if any association was demonstrated (Weich, Lewis and Jenkins 2002).

The relationship between health and other social factors is enormously complex and despite limitations in existing evidence, Richard Wilkinson raises important questions about the role of social inequality. For this to be regarded as an effective argument, not only is adequate empirical evidence required, it is also necessary to have a convincing explanation that could account for this relationship. Why should inequality in society generate inequality in health status? This is a question that Wilkinson and others have addressed, and is returned to in the next chapter, in relation to the role of wider societal relationships on our well-being. At this point, we turn to consider issues concerning the role of lifestyle factors on health.

Health and the role of lifestyle factors

The nineteenth-century satirist, Samuel Butler, wrote of an imaginary country where criminals were treated as sick, while punishment was meted out to those who were ill. One episode in the story involves the trial of a young man with consumption (tuberculosis), to which the state responds as if it were a crime. The 'prisoner' pleads not guilty to having committed a crime, claiming that the symptoms were in fact ones he was feigning:

> Counsel for the prisoner was allowed to urge everything that could be said in his defence: the line taken was that the prisoner was simulating consumption in order to defraud an insurance company, from which he was about to buy an annuity, and that he hoped thus to obtain it on more advantageous terms. If this could have been shown to be the case he would have escaped a criminal prosecution, and been sent to a hospital as for a moral ailment.
>
> (Butler 1970)

The jury eventually retires and returns to find the man guilty of having consumption, whereupon the judge delivers the sentence:

> It is all very well for you to say that you came of unhealthy parents, and had a severe accident in your childhood which permanently undermined your constitution; excuses such as these are the ordinary refuge of the criminal; but they cannot for one moment be listened to by the ear of justice. I am not here to enter upon curious metaphysical questions as to the origin of this or that – questions to which there would be no end were their introduction once tolerated, and which would result in throwing the only guilt on the tissues of the primordial cell, or on the elementary gases. There is no question of how you came to be wicked, but only this – namely, are you wicked or not? This has been decided in the affirmative, neither can I hesitate for a single moment to say that it has been decided justly...
>
> It is intolerable that an example of such terrible enormity should be allowed to go at large unpunished. Your presence in the society of respectable people would lead the less able-bodied to think more lightly of all forms of illness; neither can it be permitted that you should have the chance of corrupting unborn beings who might hereafter pester you. The unborn must not be allowed to come near you: and this not so much for their protection (for they are our natural enemies), as for our own; for since they will not be utterly gainsaid, it must be seen to that they shall be quartered upon those who are least likely to corrupt them.
>
> (Butler 1970)

Written as satire, Butler would presumably have been amazed to learn that one hundred years later a health food company in the US adopted the name, Erewhon. An explanation for this choice is provided on the company's website:

> We thought you might like to know a little of the history and background of Erewhon. We are often asked about our name. Erewhon is taken from the Utopian novel of the same name written by Samuel Butler in the 1800s about a

land where people are held responsible for their own health. Today, this seems more appropriate than ever.

(Erewhon Natural Food Market web site)

Lifestyle and public policy

The role of individual lifestyle is frequently in the forefront of public policy designed to promote better health and well-being. Recent examples have been quoted earlier, as in John Reid's speech in early 2004, but these are very much in keeping with the approach dominant for much of the past quarter century or more. In 1976, the view of the then Labour Government was presented in a consultation document on health:

> We as a society are becoming increasingly aware of how much depends on the attitudes and actions of the individual about his health ... Many of the major problems of prevention are less related to man's outside environment than to his own personal behaviour; what may be termed his lifestyle ... To a large extent, it is clear that the weight of responsibility for his own health lies on the shoulders of the individual himself.
>
> (Graham 1990: 195)

In 1987, the Conservative Government's White Paper, *Promoting Better Health*, identified lifestyle factors as a major contribution to major health problems of cancer, heart disease and obesity, concluding: 'much of this distress and suffering could be avoided if more members of the public took greater responsibility for looking after their own health' (Graham 1990: 196).

The overwhelming importance that leading politicians, and many others, attribute to lifestyle factors is remarkable when the limited empirical evidence supporting this view is considered. Margaret Whitehead, in a report published in 1992 with the title, *The Health Divide*, considers evidence on health inequalities and asks the question: how much of the differential does lifestyle explain? (Whitehead 1992: 323).

Evidence on the role of lifestyle

A considerable amount of data is described by Whitehead, including a longitudinal study conducted in Alameda County, California, since 1965. This shows that the death rate among the poorest group is more than twice that among the wealthiest group, and:

> Even when the data were adjusted to take account of thirteen known risk factors including smoking, drinking, exercise and race, there was still a substantial gradient of risk associated with income. For example, the poorest group still had one and a half times the risk of death as the richest group.
>
> (Whitehead 1992: 324)

The researchers concluded that behaviour and lifestyle were not the major factors associated with the higher risk of death. Another study referred to by Whitehead is a long-running piece of research examining coronary heart disease among London-based civil servants (frequently referred to as the Whitehall study, and its sequel, the Whitehall II study). Results show substantially higher rates of death from coronary heart disease among lower occupational grades. There is also a considerable contrast in smoking rates: 61 per cent of the lowest grade smoked, compared to 29 per cent in the top grade. Is it therefore the case that smoking is the main factor causing the grade differentials?

Apparently not, because when factors such as smoking were controlled for, the risk associated with smoking declined but only by 25 per cent. In other words, behaviours such as smoking might seem to account for perhaps one-quarter of the higher death rate among the lower grade civil servants, but around three-quarters of the excess deaths among the lower grade staff did not seem attributable to these factors.

This is an aspect that researchers involved in the Whitehall studies continue to pursue. Overall, on a simple comparison, the data that has been accumulated shows death rates among the lowest occupational grades are 1.8 times higher than for the most senior grades. Further comparisons, controlling not only for smoking but also blood pressure, plasma cholesterol, short height and blood sugar, showed the lowest occupational group still had a death rate 1.5 times higher than the senior grades. The lead researcher in the Whitehall study, Michael Marmot, notes these factors are important, but: ' "Adjusting" for these risk factors explains less than a third of the social gradient in mortality from heart disease' (Marmot 2004: 44).

Another estimate of the contribution of lifestyle factors, from a different study, suggests that between 10 and 30 per cent of the inequalities between socio-economic groups can be explained by differences in lifestyles and health-related behaviours (Lantz *et al.* 1998). Research of this kind provides valuable information about the relative contribution of different factors but it would be a mistake to assume that these operate independently of one another. From a health and lifestyle survey based on a sample of 9000 people, Blaxter (1990) demonstrates the existence of quite complex patterns of behaviour, with individuals showing a capability of adopting a mix of 'healthy' and 'unhealthy' lifestyles:

> Examination of different patterns show that few generalizations can be made about the 'protective' effect of various combinations of behaviour. These effects often differ between the young and the old, or between men and women, and are commonly more clearly related to the social characteristics of the people who are most likely to display the particular behaviour pattern.
>
> Thus a tentative conclusion can be reached: behavioural habits are certainly relevant to health, but perhaps less so than the social environment in which they are embedded.
>
> (Blaxter 1990: 202)

Debates over the relative contribution of personal lifestyles and social environment may, therefore, miss the point. As Whitehead puts it 'behaviour cannot be separated from its social context' (Whitehead 1992: 316). No sensible reading of the substantial research literature in this area can lead to any conclusion other than that lifestyle and behaviour is important for health. But it is no more important than many other factors, and is not separate from or independent of other circumstances. The degree of emphasis given to it by politicians may be misplaced.

Health: rights and responsibilities

If, as the evidence suggests, there is a tendency to disproportionately focus on the contribution of individual lifestyle and behaviour factors, this has considerable relevance in the context of current debates about the relationship between rights and responsibilities. Edward Peck draws attention to connections between apparently unconnected examples:

> There was media outrage when the ex-footballer George Best started drinking again following his liver transplant. Meanwhile, the government faced widespread condemnation by proposing to give psychiatrists powers to medicate mentally ill people in the community. A man was sent to prison for knowingly infecting his sexual partners with the HIV virus. The Labour Party has suggested we should sign agreements with our GP committing us, for example, to give up smoking or take more exercise.
>
> Four seemingly unrelated issues, but the link is that each illustrates one of the arguments that might be used to further extend the obligations that we have to take care of our own health or to use health services more responsibly. The government seems ready to extend the ideas about rights and responsibilities that have informed other areas of public policy.
>
> (Guardian 25.08.04)

Nor is it politicians alone who raise these issues. Writing of experiences working in an inner-city NHS hospital, one doctor objected to proposals by the National Institute for Clinical Excellence that NHS staff should be better trained in dealing with people who self-harm:

> It strikes me that the people who hurt themselves deliberately, or who try to kill themselves and then come to hospital seeking help, are the victims of many wrongs – bad relationships, unemployment, poverty, mental illness and addictions – but they are not the victims of bad healthcare. They get their wounds stitched, their overdoses treated and a psychiatric review, time and again. They get kindness and endless patience from tired, busy staff ...
>
> Self-harmers who attend hospital habitually are unable to take responsibility for their own lives and actions, and it might be that by being so patient and non-judgemental we are fostering that destructive cycle.
>
> (Guardian 03.08.04)

There is a certain symmetry between these remarks and the analysis offered by critics of medicine, such as Ivan Illich. This is in terms of questioning whether problems faced by people in coping with their lives are best resolved by turning to the health care system. The question relates back to the debate on how far professionals should seek involvement in aspects of the patient's life beyond the clinical issues. That aspect aside, the examples above raise another important issue.

This concerns a tendency to seek explanations for personal behaviour in individualistic terms. This can be especially true for politicians, however, for professionals, too, this can seem to provide a ready answer. Our capacity to act as autonomous individuals is not unbounded: this is why understanding the social context of individual behaviour is so important.

The subsequent two chapters develop this theme by exploring psychosocial influences on health and illness. Chapter 8 considers this by examining the role of social support and social networks, from those of family and community to wider societal relationships. In Chapter 9 attention moves to examining issues arising in employment and work relationships. The objective is to help develop a way of thinking about individual experiences that roots them within the social settings in which they arise.

8
Society, relationships and health

Late in the summer of 2004, under the title 'The Death of Intimacy', an article in the *Guardian* newspaper sketched a bleak view of the quality of contemporary human relationships:

> Recent surveys indicating that we are less happy than we used to be suggest a profound malaise at the heart of western society and modern notions of progress ... The reason we no longer feel as happy as we once did is that the intimacy on which our sense of well-being rests – a product of our closest, most intimate relationships, above all in the family – is in decline.
>
> *(Guardian* 18.09.04)

If this assessment is accurate there are considerable implications for how we interpret the nation's state of health. For there is evidence to suggest that the quality of our relationships has a substantial effect on our health, with stronger social networks seemingly associated with less illness. In addition, these networks have consequences for how we cope with illness and disability. Attention is given to these issues in this chapter, in three stages: the role of intimate and confiding relationships; community relations; and wider societal relationships. This is done purely as a means of organizing the material, not to suggest these are three separate and distinct spheres.

Intimacy and confiding relationships

Brown and Harris' research examining the social origins of depression among women has been referred to as an example of a study seeking to understand individual experiences in their social context. One aspect that interested Brown and Harris was the role of social support, and having reviewed some of the literature on this at that time (1978) they observed:

> Sidney Cobb (1976) has recently undertaken a broad review of the socio-medical literature for any suggestion that social support acts to prevent ill health. The studies are a mixed bag and evidence rather poor but his review is

enough to suggest that support may play a role in mediating between stress and other forms of disorder.

(Brown and Harris 1979: 178–9)

Two specific studies are referred to: one showing that women without social support were more likely to experience complications in pregnancy following some kind of life crisis; and the second indicating that men with low levels of social support were more likely to develop arthritic symptoms after experiencing a loss of their job. From their own research data Brown and Harris concluded that intimacy was an important factor influencing how women coped with problems that might trigger depression. Emotional rather than sexual intimacy was involved: 'We found that if a woman does not have an intimate tie, someone she can trust and confide in, particularly a husband or boyfriend, she is much more likely to break down in the presence of a severe event or major difficulty' (Brown and Harris 1979: 278).

They later remark:

The role of social isolation in depression is also suggested by the ability of an intimate relationship to reduce risk of disorder. While such a relationship is likely to help provide some women with a basic sense of self-worth it also has its more active aspect. The availability of a confidant, a person to whom one can reveal one's weaknesses without risk of rebuff and thus further loss of self-esteem, may act as a buttress against the total evaporation of feelings of self-worth following a major loss or disappointment.

(Brown and Harris 1979: 286)

The conclusion that intimate relationships play an important role in our health receives support from a study of nearly 8000 London-based civil servants. The study is described in greater detail elsewhere. However, one finding was that having intimate and confiding relationships were important predictors of mental health, but with differences between men and women. For men, low levels of confiding and of emotional support were associated with greater risks of psychiatric morbidity, whereas for women, emotional support was associated with good mental health but this was not the case if confiding opportunities were present alone. Negative aspects of close relationships predicted poor mental health for both men and women (Stansfield, Fuhrer and Shipley 1998).

As always, caution is needed in interpreting results showing a correlation between two different factors. Direct causal associations cannot be assumed. For example, one study of 600 people in Manchester who had experienced a heart attack found considerable differences between those with and those without an intimate relationship. Results showed that those without someone close whom they could confide in were twice as likely to have another heart attack within a year as those having such a person. The study took account of factors such as age, history of heart disease and the severity of the original attack. However, it is possible that the quality of intimate relationships has only an indirect effect. For example, those without a close relationship were more likely to drink heavily and use illegal drugs. Nevertheless, Belinda Linden, the head of medical information at the British Heart

Foundation, which part-funded the study with the Medical Research Council, commented:

> A close relationship, whether it be lover, friend or relative, is obviously a potentially vital source of social support, which can play an important role in both preventing coronary heart disease and enhancing recovery from attack.
>
> (*Guardian* 15.04.04)

Changing relationships

Historically, the institution of marriage has provided a major route into establishing and maintaining intimacy, and the decline of marriage has been one of the most significant social changes in the latter part of the twentieth century. In 1941–5, 71 per cent of men and 68 per cent of women aged over 15 years were married, but by 1991–5 the comparable figures were 36 per cent and 44 per cent (Coleman 2000). However, the growing number of people choosing to cohabit without entering into the legal relationship of marriage limits the value of this data for making accurate assessments about changes taking place.

An alternative source of data for this question is provided by a series of three studies conducted in Britain since 1946. These have tracked the experiences of everyone born in a single week in the years 1946, 1958 and 1970, producing a unique picture of changes during this time. A summary of the overall research project observed:

> One of the most striking changes across the period was in attitudes and behaviour towards relationships and the postponement of the commitments involved in marriage and parenthood.
>
> (Ferri, Bynner and Wadsworth 2003: 4)

One study within this research project focused on changes in partnerships and parenthood. It found:

> For example, 77 per cent of men and 88 per cent of women born in 1946 were married by the age of 31, twice as many as among the 1970 cohort. Cohabitation was virtually unreported by those born in 1946, whereas a third of those born in 1958 were living with partners to whom they were not married by the time they were 30.
>
> (Ferri and Smith 2003)

Even with rising divorce rates, cohabitation is less likely to result in a permanent relationship than is marriage, and so it seems very likely that an increasing number of adults will experience a series of intimate relationships, rather than maintain a single one. There may be consequences of this for wider family relationships, particularly where children are involved, but a shift towards serial monogamy, as it is sometimes described, provides no indication of what is happening to the quality of intimate relationships.

A question asked of the 1958 and 1970 cohorts, but not of the 1946 group, was 'How happy is your relationship with your spouse or partner?' Among men born in 1958, 3 per cent of those married for the first time and 2 per cent of those married for the second time described themselves as being unhappy at age 33 (in 1991). The proportion was 1 per cent among those who were cohabiting. The equivalent figures for women describing themselves as being in 'unhappy' relationships were 2 per cent for both those married for the first time and second time and 6 per cent of those cohabiting.

Comparing these results with those for people born in 1970 reveals some substantial differences. Twenty-two per cent of men married for the first time and 18 per cent of those married for a second time and cohabiting described their relationship as 'unhappy' at age 30 (in 2000). For women the equivalent figures were 24 per cent, 21 per cent and 20 per cent. This suggests a remarkably high level of dissatisfaction among those born more recently. One suggestion has been that younger people in today's society have unrealistic expectations about relationships, resulting in a much greater likelihood that they will be dissatisfied and disappointed. This view appears to have gained popular currency, illustrated in remarks by Naomi Harris, the 27-year-old actress who appeared in the film 28 Days Later:

> I think our problem is that we have so much choice now that people flounder a lot more because they don't know what decision to take. We are never quite satisfied in a relationship because we always think we might get something better and we are never willing to settle.
>
> (*Sunday Telegraph* 20.06.04)

The title of the *Sunday Telegraph* article in which that comment appeared, 'Unhappy with their life, work and love – that's Britain's 30-year-olds', deliberately suggests a generational change in attitudes towards relationships. However, an alternative interpretation is suggested by responses to the question about happiness in relationships from members of the 1958 cohort, when aged 42 in 2000. Despite giving generally very positive descriptions of their relationships in 1991, nine years later their responses were much closer to those of the 1970 cohort. For men, 19 per cent of those married for the first time, 17 per cent of those married for the second time and 13 per cent of those cohabiting described their relationship as 'unhappy'. For women, the figures were 20 per cent, 21 per cent and 15 per cent.

Yet another explanation could be that there is an 'age effect', with relationships becoming less satisfying as time goes on. If this is the case, it suggests some very high levels of dissatisfaction are likely among younger groups as they move into middle age.

Although the 1946 cohort were not asked questions about the happiness of their relationships, data on their divorce rates is available. By 1978, when aged 31, just 2 per cent of men and 3 per cent of women had been divorced or separated. But by their early 40s, 12 per cent of men and 16 per cent of the women were no longer living in a partnership.

More analysis of this data is required to explore the factors that may be associated with unhappy relationships, although initial examination suggests less positive relationships are slightly more likely among women who became mothers by age 30, among men who had partnered very young, and among both men and women in partnerships where neither was in employment (Ferri and Smith 2003: 116).

However, early observations by those working with this data signal an important trend:

> One of the most striking findings to emerge from the comparisons described in this chapter relates to the growing fragility of personal relationships. Each successive cohort reveals an increasing instability in marriage and cohabitation . . .
>
> . . . Further analysis will be needed to try and account for the relative disillusionment with personal relationships among the 1970 cohort at 30 – and among the 1958 cohort as they entered middle age. For example, to what extent is it linked to the pressures on relationships created by competing demands of employment and domestic roles? Whatever the explanation, the apparent growth in negative perceptions of personal relationships, together with the increasing impermanence of partnerships, both married and cohabiting, can be seen as indicative of uncertainty and insecurity permeating family life in Britain at the start of the twenty-first century.
>
> (Ferri and Smith 2003: 131–2)

Hidden suffering

These are important developments, but it would be a gross error to assume that greater permanency of relationships in the past was any guarantee of their quality. Only three decades ago, in 1975, a Parliamentary Select Committee published a report, 'Violence in Marriage', that included an extract from evidence submitted by the Association of Chief Police Constables:

> It is important to keep 'wife battering' in its correct perspective and realise that this loose term is applied to incidents ranging from a very minor domestic fracas where no Police action is really justified, to the more serious incidents of assaults occasioning grievous bodily harm and unlawful woundings. Whilst such problems take up considerable Police time during, say, 12 months, in the majority of cases the role of the Police is a negative one. We are, after all, dealing with persons 'bound in marriage', and it is important for a host of reasons, to maintain the unity of the spouses.
>
> (Quoted in Pahl 1985)

Not until the 1990s did the British courts accept that rape was possible within marriage. Prior to then it was assumed that marriage gave rights of sexual pleasure to the male, regardless of the woman's wishes. In 1972 the soft pornography magazine, *Penthouse*, challenged attempts by the nascent feminist movement to bring the issue of rape into the spotlight of public concern. In one example, the magazine asserted that rape could not occur because sexual intercourse always required consent: 'it is virtually impossible for a woman to be sexually penetrated *against her will* by a single, unaided man' (*Penthouse* 1972, cited in Collins 2003).

Welcome changes in attitudes have occurred since then and it may be that the abuse and suffering that past arrangements were capable of concealing are no longer accepted in the same way. The evidence of unhappiness in contemporary personal relationships is nevertheless important, and should be heeded, but also needs to be considered in the context of wider community developments. If it is true that personal relationships are becoming less satisfying, what of wider social networks?

Social relationships and community

Beyond our close, confiding partnerships are others that may involve less intimacy but nevertheless count amongst our most important. Although different in kind to the closer intimacy of a personal relationship, these wider relationships also act as significant sources of social support. The importance of these relationships has been emphasized by Robert Putnam who, in his book, *Bowling Alone*, makes the claim that of all the domains he investigated: 'in none is the importance of social connectedness so well established as in the case of health and illness' (Putnam 2000: 326).

There is a substantial range of work that supports this conclusion. A review of over 50 studies examining the association between social support and cardiovascular function reported that individuals with high levels of social support had lower blood pressure than individuals with lower levels of social support (Uchino 1999). The presence of social support may also reduce the negative effects of a stressful experience. One study, in which individuals were exposed to the stress of participating in a debate, typically found this to be associated with raised blood pressure and increased heart rate. However, when accompanied by someone who agreed with their position, the scale of these changes was reduced (Gerin, Pieper, Levy and Pickering 1992).

Social networks also appear to reduce the risk of infection from the common cold. In one study, participants were exposed to common-cold viruses, via nasal drops, and then quarantined for five days: 'Individuals who had more diverse social networks (i.e. relationships in a variety of domains, such as work, home and church) were less likely to develop clinical colds than individuals with less diverse networks' (Putnam 2000).

Much of the research in this area appears to justify the conclusion reached by Putnam:

Social networks help you stay healthy ... As a rule of thumb, if you belong to no groups but decide to join one, you cut your risk of dying over the next year *in half*. If you smoke and belong to no groups, it's a toss-up statistically whether you should stop smoking or start joining. These findings are in some ways heartening; it's easier to join a group than to lose weight, exercise regularly, or quit smoking.

(Putnam 2000: 331)

The nature of community

The role of social networks has long been a key topic of interest for sociology, traditionally reflected in the concept of community:

'Community' stands as a convenient shorthand term for the broad realm of social arrangements beyond the private sphere of home and family but more familiar to us than the impersonal institutions of the wider society, what Bulmer calls 'intermediary structures'. The diversity and spread of these structures helps to account for the bewildering variety of meanings associated with the term 'community'. Community ties may be structured around links between people with common residence, common interests, common attachments or some other shared experience generating a sense of belonging.

(Crow and Allan 1994: 1)

The precise form that a community takes can vary greatly. It may be based upon a geographical locality or a lifestyle, an occupation, or some other interest or involvement. Place, as in a neighbourhood, provides an important source for community ties but by no means the only one. The key feature is that community provides a unit of involvement to which we can relate and engage in. As an opportunity to escape the 'impersonal institutions of the wider society', location continues to provide an important source of experiences that we share with those around us.

People may be less firmly rooted in the neighbourhood from which they came but the continuing importance of place should not be underestimated. It is a sobering thought to reflect on the fact that a black 15-year-old in Harlem or from the South Side of Chicago has about a one in three chance of reaching the age of 65. As one commentator noted:

There is something about living in these areas that takes a toll on people, people we think of as perfectly innocent, people who are just living their lives and yet are getting really sick. When people talk about men in the central cities not pulling their weight – the fact that two-thirds of them are likely to be dead before they complete their productive years I think is something people have missed.

(Geronimus *et al.* 1996)

The importance of place

Evidence from England and Wales also points to the importance of place, with one study noting that alongside social class inequalities in health, 'the health of people in each social class varied considerably depending on where they lived' (Doran, Drever and Whitehead 2004: 1043).

The data shows 75 people per 1000 in routine occupations living in the East of England reporting their health as being 'not good', compared to 113 per 1000 working in similar occupations but living in Wales. People living in the South-East had better health than the British average for their own social class. This also applied to most social classes in the South-West and the East. Other examples demonstrate similar points, summed up by the authors:

> Even for people in the same social class, their risks of poor health varied greatly depending on where they lived. Women in class 1 (higher managerial and professional occupations) in Wales fared worse than women in class 4 (small employers and own account workers) in the South West, and men in class 4 in the North West fared worse than men in class 7 (routine occupations) in the South East.
>
> (Doran, Drever and Whitehead 2004: 1044)

The sociologist Richard Sennett suggests place may be becoming of increasing significance for people's sense of identity. Linking changes in the workplace with those occurring in neighbourhood and community identity, Sennett (1998) argues that many workplaces are becoming more insecure and uncertain, with an absence of trust and with only superficial team relationships. The promotion of a fear of 'failure' 'impels people to look for some other scene of attachment and depth', and this may be sought in their locality. But, Sennett warns, 'the desire for community is defensive, often expressed as rejection of immigrants or other outsiders' (Sennett 1998: 138).

Outsiders and the established

This picks up on an important theme, one addressed in research conducted in the 1960s by Norbert Elias (1965/1994). Elias studied relationships within a small community, Winston Parva, in which there was a significant segregation between the 'established' and the 'outsiders'. He observed:

> a sharp division within it between an old-established group and a newer group of residents, whose members were treated as outsiders by the established group. The latter closed ranks and stigmatized them generally as people of lesser human worth. They were thought to lack the superior human virtue – the distinguishing group charisma – which the dominant group attributed to itself.
>
> (Elias and Scotson 1994: xv)

There was no difference of nationality, ethnic origin, or even occupation and social class between the two groups: 'Both were working class areas. The only difference between them was that mentioned before: one group was formed by old residents established in the neighbourhood for two or three generations and the other was a group of newcomers' (Elias and Scotson 1994: xvii).

Community, as writers such as Putnam accept, is not always a positive experience. Inclusion for some can mean exclusion for others. Place is an important aspect of community but our most significant relationships can be a complex blend. Sometimes this may incorporate place, family and friendships, a point raised in research on the family in the 1950s by Elizabeth Bott, who concluded:

> The immediate social environment of urban families is best considered not as the local area in which they live, but rather as the network of actual social relationships they maintain, regardless of whether these are confined to the local area or run beyond its boundaries.

> (Bott 1957: 99)

Teenage motherhood: the role of family and community

Family relationships have changed dramatically in the half century since Elizabeth Bott was writing but in many settings the interrelated influences of family and community continue to have a considerable effect. A demonstration of this comes in a study of decisions by young women about whether or not to proceed with a pregnancy (Lee, Clements, Ingham and Stone 2004). This revealed decisions to be subject to a range of social and cultural attitudes and expectations.

Between 1999 and 2001 44 per cent of conceptions among 15–17-year-olds were terminated. However, this average conceals wide local variations. Rates in individual local authorities range from 18 per cent in Derwentside, County Durham, to 76 per cent in Eden, Cumbria. As there can also be considerable variation within a local authority, the scale of difference between different areas of the country can be substantial.

Using interviews with 103 teenagers, as well as statistical data, the study found that decisions about abortions were generally made before visiting a health professional. The existence of such divergent outcomes therefore prompts questions about the factors that may lie behind them. How do young women reach a decision about whether or not to proceed with the pregnancy?

An obvious assumption might be to begin by considering moral or religious beliefs, given the importance these have for defining attitudes towards the acceptability or otherwise of terminating a pregnancy. However, it was not generally these that were found to be the more important determinant of outcome. Instead: 'decision-making appeared to be influenced by their socio-economic circumstances, family and community views and availability of services'. (Lee *et al.* 2004: 48.)

An important aspect was the consequences that social and family circumstances had for expectations and aspirations for the future: 'Those who opted for abortion tended to have high expectations of life in the present, and clear pathways marked out for the immediate future'. (Report summary)

Young women who anticipated entering higher education were much more likely to proceed with a termination, as illustrated in the following extract from an interview: 'There was no question of me keeping it because I knew I was going to go to university . . . I'd had a good education and I had a career path to go down, it was all laid out for me.' (p. 18)

For young women such as these, motherhood was something to be delayed. Independence from the responsibilities of child care was seen as essential to achieve their aims and ambitions. Young women for whom such plans did not exist and who neither sought nor expected a future of this kind, were far more likely to adopt a positive view of motherhood. Even if a pregnancy had not been planned or expected, it was less likely to be seen as a major impediment to future plans.

In some cases, quite the opposite occurred, with young women referring to the experience of becoming a mother in very positive terms: 'It has been the best thing that's ever happened to me . . . if I hadn't had the baby I'm sure I would've been in jail.' (p. 18)

Alongside the role of hopes and expectations for the future, other influences on decisions included community and family views, and experiences about motherhood. These included 'the extent to which having children relatively early was accepted and seen as normal' and 'differing perceptions of the difficulties and demands that parenthood carries with it'. (p. 49)

Analysis of abortion statistics indicates that the ratio of rates of termination among younger women tend to be relatively constant with those for older women. In other words, although the rates vary between different age groups, within local areas there appears to be some consistency between them. Rates are higher among younger women in places where they are also higher among older women. Again, this suggests a role being played by local family and community influences.

Many of the young women who continued with their pregnancy reported that other members of the family, particularly female members, played an important role, often helping out with child care arrangements. This was frequently the case for those who described abortion as being 'wrong', as in the words of one young woman: 'My Mum will never have an abortion and she hasn't made up my mind for me, but she was always that way.' (p. 44)

Another recalled: 'I was kind of hoping for her to say: "Well you're young, get rid of it." There was a lot of pressure for me to keep him' (Lee, Clements, Ingham and Stone 2004: 43).

Family and kinship relationships in many close-knit communities have been subject to enormous change for several years. Often this has been associated with the closure of traditional sources of employment. This can create feelings of isolation, however, other forms of social relationships can develop in the place of those being eroded. Friendships are particularly important, reminding us of the need to consider the quality of relationships, rather than the precise form they take at a particular point in time. There can be many negative consequences of changes that occur but historical examples illustrate how adaptable humans can be.

Community and association

Links between physical location, social relationships and personal characteristics have long been seen to exist. More than a century and a half ago, Benjamin Disraeli claimed the growth of cities was creating more than a harmful physical environment:

> In great cities men are brought together by the desire of gain. They are not in a state of co-operation, but of isolation, as to the making of fortunes; and for all the rest they are careless of neighbours. Christianity teaches us to love our neighbour as ourself; modern society acknowledges no neighbour.
>
> (Cited in Putnam 2000: 380)

From that time on, numerous commentators bemoaned the loss of community brought by the processes of urbanization. Of particular prominence was the German writer, Ferdinand Tonnies, who contrasted social relationships existing in the pre-industrial and industrial worlds. The first – *Gemeinschaft* – is normally translated as 'community' and was characterized by close, enduring relationships, in which the roles of different individuals were clearly defined and understood. Such communities also tended to be quite fixed, with little movement in or out of them.

Industrial society was characterized by a different type of relationship – *Gessellschaft* – which is often translated as 'association'. This involves much weaker, impersonal relationships between people; calculative and contractual rather than close and enduring.

One of the most striking contributions to the examination of the impact of urban and industrial society upon social relationships came from another German, George Simmel. In a piece of work, 'The Metropolis and Mental Life', in 1902, Simmel contrasts the 'intensification of nervous stimulation' that occurs in the large town with: 'small town life which rests more upon deeply felt and emotional relationships'.

The metropolis, argues Simmel, requires intellectual rather than emotional involvement, and with this comes a stronger emphasis on the importance of money and economic relationships. Human associations transform from emotional into rational relationships: 'All intimate emotional relations between persons are founded in their individuality, whereas in rational relations man is reckoned with like a number, like an element which is in itself indifferent' (Cited in Thompson and Tunstall 1971: 83–4).

Emphasizing the anonymity of the city, with increasing numbers of people having to integrate their activities into a highly complex organism, he sees this creating what he describes as a 'blasé attitude'. By this he means people respond to excessive stimulation by treating things as if they are insubstantial. There are, he believed, accompanying changes in responses to other people. With so many contacts there is a tendency to adopt 'reserve':

> If so many inner reactions were responses to the continuous external contacts with innumerable people as are those in the small town, where one knows

almost everybody one meets and where one has a positive relation to almost everyone, one would be completely atomized internally and come to an unimaginable psychic state. Partly this psychological fact, partly the right to distrust which men have in the face of the touch-and-go elements of metropolitan life, necessitates our reserve. As a result of this reserve we frequently do not even know by sight those who have been our neighbour for years.

(Cited in Thompson and Tunstall 1971: 88)

With this, Simmel suggests, comes a level of personal freedom previously unknown in human society:

The earliest phase of social formation found in historical as well as contemporary social structures is this: a relatively small circle firmly closed against neighbouring, strange or in some way antagonistic circles. However, this circle is closely coherent and allows its individual members only a narrow field for the development of unique qualities and free, self-responsible movements.

(Cited in Thompson and Tunstall 1971: 88–9)

People living in the city are no longer subject to the 'pettiness and prejudice which hem in the small-town man'. However, the freedom this escape allows also means that: 'one nowhere feels as lonely and lost as in the metropolitan crowd'.

One good reason for reading Simmel today is to benefit from his insights into social change, but another is to indicate how laments for a loss of community are not only a feature of contemporary society. This perception of modern society, as one in which human contacts are fleeting and transitory, was prompted by urban growth that itself later became the site of strong communities. Compare Disraeli's remarks on urbanization in the mid-nineteenth century with the following extracts from a study of the East End of London in the 1950s:

As she went along the street, nodding and chatting to this person and that, Mrs Landon commented on the people whom she saw.

Mary Collins: 'She's a sister of Sally who I worked with at the button place before I got married. My Mum knew her Mum, but I sort of lost touch until one day I found myself sitting next to her in Meath gardens. We both had the babies with us and so we got talking again. I see quite a lot of Mary now.'

Mavis Boot: 'That lady there, I know her. She lives down our turning,' said Mrs Landon, as she caught sight in the butcher's of a back view of a large woman carrying the usual flat cloth bag. 'She's the daughter of one of Mum's old friends. When she died Mum promised to keep an eye on Mavis. She pops in at Mum's every day.'

Sadie Little: This time there was not even a nod. The two women walked straight past each other. 'She's quarrelled with my sister so we don't talk to each other.'

Violet Belcher: a tall, thin lady talking to another at the street corner is, 'an acquaintance of Mum's. She's got trouble with her insides.'

She kept a record over a week of all the people she saw in the street and whom she considered herself to 'know'. There were sixty-three people in all, some seen many times and thirty-eight of them relatives of at least one other person out of the sixty-three. Her story showed how she had built up a series of connections with people she had known in school, work or street and even more forcefully, how her mother and other kin acted as a means of communication between herself and the other people in her social world.

(Young and Willmott 1957: 82–4)

This community grew in urban locations that had earlier been condemned for destroying genuine human association. Yet, despite the evidence of strong social attachment, the health of many people living in such communities was often poor. How, then, can the relationship between health and community be understood?

Social cohesion and health

This is a question considered by Richard Wilkinson, as part of his analysis of the statistical association between inequalities in wealth and inequalities in health. An example both he and Robert Putnam use to support their arguments is drawn from Roseto in Pennsylvania, a small town with a population of around 1600. The town attracted interest from researchers because of its very low mortality rates, particularly from heart attacks. Death rates had been lower than neighbouring areas since the 1930s, about 40 per cent lower in the case of heart disease, and research suggested that this could not be accounted for by factors such as diet, smoking and exercise.

Instead, the explanation seemed to lie in the particular social history of the town. Made up largely of descendants of migrants from the Italian town of Roseto, it became evident to the researchers that the town continued to be characterized by 'close family ties and cohesive community relations' (Egolf et al. 1992: 1089).

The researchers also noted:

During the first five years of our study it was difficult to distinguish, on the basis of dress or behaviour, the wealthy from the impecunious in Roseto. Living arrangements – houses and cars – were simple and strikingly similar. Despite the affluence of many, there was no atmosphere of 'keeping up with the Joneses'.

(Bruhn and Wolf 1979: 81–2)

From the beginning the sense of common purpose and the camaraderie among the Italians precluded ostentation or embarrassment to the less affluent, and the concern for neighbors ensured that no one was ever abandoned. This pattern of remarkable social cohesion, in which the family, as the hub and bulwark of life, provided a kind of security and insurance against any catastrophe, was associated with the striking absence of myocardial infarction and sudden death.

(Bruhn and Wolf 1979: 136)

The concept of social capital

Both Wilkinson and Putnam believe that evidence such as this points to the importance of 'social capital':

> Social capital refers to connections among individuals – social networks and the norms of reciprocity and trustworthiness that arise from them. In that sense social capital is closely related to what some have called 'civic virtue'. The difference is that 'social capital' calls attention to the fact that civic virtue is most powerful when embedded in a dense network of reciprocal social relations. A society of many virtuous but isolated individuals is not necessarily rich in social capital.
>
> (Putnam 2000: 19)

The idea of 'reciprocal social relations' is at the heart of the notion of social capital. Recent years have seen a burgeoning literature around this theme, not least in relation to its possible association with health status. The approach has also been adopted by many leading politicians, including the British Prime Minister, Tony Blair:

> As Robert Putnam argues ... communities that are inter-connected are healthier communities. If we play football together, run parent–teacher associations together, sing in choirs or learn to paint together, we are less likely to want to cause harm to each other. Such inter-connected communities have lower crime, better education results, better care of the vulnerable. Governments can support communities indirectly, by letting go of power for example, or by providing good public services, which cut crime, improve education or transport.
>
> (Blair 2002: 12–13)

Putnam (2000) suggests four possible explanations for this association. First, social networks can provide practical means of support, such as giving a lift to a clinic appointment, or someone to notice if you have not been out for a day or so. Second, social networks may provide support for healthy norms, whereas damaging behaviours, such as heavy drinking or smoking, may be more frequent among socially isolated individuals. Third, communities that are socially cohesive may be more successful in gaining better facilities, including health care, that promote better health. Fourth, 'and most intriguingly, social capital might actually serve as a physiological triggering mechanism, stimulating people's immune systems to fight disease and buffer stress' (Putnam 2000: 327).

Whatever might be the explanation, Putnam and others argue that social capital has been in decline in countries such as the US. Not everyone supports this assessment. Robert Wuthnow, for example, emphasizes the need to accept that the form of civil involvement will change and that new styles are emerging. Without denying the existence of problems surrounding levels of community involvement, Wuthnow argues:

Although the demise of civil society is a spectre that has alarmed many social observers, a close look at civil involvement today reveals that many Americans still care deeply about their communities and make efforts to connect with other people. But these efforts generally do not take the same forms as they had in the past because of the increased diversity, fluidity, independence, and specialization of contemporary life. The new, loosely structured forms of civic involvement often leave people with the sense that they are not doing enough to help others and that their communities are coming apart at the seams.

Of course there are serious problems in our society, such as crime, homelessness and domestic violence, and these problems could be addressed more effectively if more Americans became involved in community organizations and took a more active interest in political affairs. Yet the main difficulty in generating greater civic engagement is not some moral malaise but rather a profound change in the character of our institutions. Whereas earlier conventions and ways of life created well-defined roles that tended to characterize and restrict people for their entire lives, today's more flexible roles create institutions that allow for and even require more negotiation and change. In the process of adjusting to these new institutional realities, we have had to invent new ways of being involved in our communities.

(Wuthnow 1998: 203)

Rejecting the more pessimistic accounts of some writers, Wuthnow points to the importance of people's sense of involvement. He argues this is under strain more owing to changes in the institutions through which it can be achieved, rather than because of a more fundamental loss of a sense of belonging. This could still, presumably, have negative consequences for health but historical experiences of changes in society and community should alert us to the danger of assuming too readily that these represent its demise.

The growth of self-help groups

An example of a newer form of social engagement might be the emergence of self-help groups, many of which have developed around issues of health or disability. Groups of this type represent a form of association that has been increasing, in Britain, Europe and the US (Kelleher 1994). A number of studies indicate that belonging to a support group can have beneficial consequences for recovery. In a study of breast cancer patients, those who were randomly assigned to a support group were found to live almost twice as long as those who received routine oncological care without participation in the support group.

A review of literature in this area refers to work on social support and coronary artery disease, depressive symptoms, diabetes, Alzheimer's disease, Parkinson's disease and sickle cell syndromes: 'While little is known about how support affects illness or changes in health status, research has shown that a lack of social support has been associated with increased mortality risk, delay from recovery from disease, poor morale and poor mental health' (White and Cant 2003: 329).

Similarly, a pilot study into the role of social support networks, conducted among 30 HIV-positive gay men in Greater London suggests that social support networks played a major role in the lives of these men. Although numbers involved in the study were small, the networks were found to provide important sources of instrumental and emotional support, involving partners, ex-partners and friends. Few of the men described themselves as being estranged from their families but these were not the main providers of social support. Nor was the 'community', in the sense of locality, cited as a source of support:

> Most of those who rejected the idea of community altogether had very strong views on the ways in which traditional communities had rejected them or expressed hostility to them on account of their sexuality or HIV status. Those who saw themselves as belonging to a community cited communities which had, for the most part, been created by their own current members.
>
> (White and Cant 2003: 332)

Examples of this kind might lend support to Wuthnow's contention that the institutional opportunities for engagement are as important as individual motivation. If so, this suggests a potential role for health professionals in stimulating opportunities for this kind of involvement.

Related to this, one final aspect of the role of social networks to note is that their absence may increase levels of demand for professional support. Research evidence exists to suggest that people without networks of social relationships or social support are more likely to be users of the health care system. In part, this is interpreted as the consequence of individuals experiencing distress, but lacking close friends or other sources of social support, being more likely to seek professional help than those with such support.

This question was explored in a community survey conducted in Baltimore, Maryland, USA, which confirmed this finding and concluded: 'Social support can be obtained in informal networks or by visits to physicians' (Kouzis and Eaton 1998: 1307). It also observed that: 'In situations where emotional social support is available, the urgency of the symptom can be assessed by comparison with another person who may not be under such a high level of stress' (Kouzis and Eaton 1998: 1308).

As was noted earlier, in spite of the decline in many traditional sources of support, new forms are emerging. But those around us do not only play an important role in providing such support: our individual behaviour is also significantly affected by the attitudes of others. This connects not just with the extent to which we feel part of a community but to a wider sense of belonging to society.

Wider societal relationships

An important aspect of our sense of belonging to society can be our willingness to behave according to prevailing social norms. Political and media attention on the issue of 'anti-social behaviour' has brought this issue very much to the fore. The normative influence that societies have upon individuals, and situations in which this may break down, was a key point of interest for the French sociologist, Emil Durkheim. His work can be approached through the analysis of health inequalities put forward by Richard Wilkinson.

In his work on health inequality, Wilkinson argues that societies with wider inequalities in health also tend to have wider inequalities in income. Acknowledging that societies with a more equal distribution of income may possess 'a more egalitarian ethic' to begin with, which might independently encourage a stronger sense of social cohesion, he asserts that for societies to develop and maintain social cohesion: 'a narrow distribution of income is a necessary condition for their survival and is likely to serve as a marker for important characteristics of the social fabric' (Wilkinson 1996: 135).

He develops his case to argue:

> Instead of merely market or self-interested relations between families and households, it appears that in more egalitarian societies the public sphere of life remains a more social sphere than it does elsewhere. It remains dominated by people's involvement in the social, ethical and human life of the society, rather than being abandoned to market values and transactions.
>
> (Wilkinson 1996: 136)

Wilkinson seems to be suggesting that societies in which income inequalities are wide are ones where individuals are more self-interested, concentrating on pursuing personal goals rather than engaging in wider community and civil activity. This would imply that income inequality has an indirect effect on health, by undermining the quality of social relationships and social cohesion.

The role of social norms

There is, though, a slightly different way in which this association might be interpreted. For this we can draw upon the work of Emil Durkheim, beginning with some of his remarks on the role of social norms:

> The totality of beliefs and sentiments common to the average members of a society forms a determinate system with a life of its own. It can be termed the collective or common consciousness ... Individuals pass on, but it abides. It is the same in north and south, in large towns and in small, and in different professions. Likewise it does not change with every generation but, on the contrary, links successive generations to each other. Thus it is something totally different from the consciousness of individuals, although it is only realized in individuals ... Thus ... we may state that an act is criminal when it offends the strong, well-defined states of the collective consciousness.
>
> (Durkheim 1997: 38–9)

Central to Durkheim's thinking was the idea that collective moral codes become necessary as human progress allows us to escape biological constraints.

Other constraints must take their place, and social restraints are substituted for those of Nature.

An important element of Durkheim's thinking is the concept of 'anomie'. Briefly, anomie can be defined as 'a social condition characterized by the break-down of norms governing social interaction' (Abercrombie, Hall and Turner 1984: 21). Durkheim's concept of anomie was, like Marx's concept of alienation to be discussed in the next chapter, intended to help understand the connections between social systems and individual experiences. Both concepts, in that sense, have the potential to help us develop a sociological imagination, connecting 'public issues' and 'private troubles'.

Confusion can sometimes arise because Durkheim used the word anomie in slightly different ways. In two of his major works, *The Division of Labour* and *Suicide*, the concept is not used with complete consistency, and while the detail of this need not concern us, a distinction drawn by Lee and Newby (1983) is worth noting. First, anomie relates to the absence of effective social regulation and rules: this is regarded as leading to inadequate coordination across society. Second, Durkheim uses the concept to describe the consequences of this state of affairs for individuals, 'producing a sense of the isolation and meaninglessness of life and work' (Lee and Newby 1983: 221). In other words, sometimes the term is used to describe a state of society and on other occasions, the condition of the individual. But, aside from this, it is important to emphasize how Durkheim saw and interpreted the individual consequences very much as the outcome of the social setting.

For Durkheim, circumstances arise that weaken the effectiveness of social norms in their ability to regulate individual behaviour. This in turn creates a state of anomie, characterized by a deregulation of social behaviour, disorientating individual appetites and desires. Individual behaviour is no longer controlled by public opinion and maintained within the limits this imposes.

Durkheim on suicide

The relationship of this argument to debates about health and inequality can be explored by considering Durkheim's study of suicide. This is a classic study, although it has received criticism from a number of directions. Some of these raise very fundamental points, such as the extent to which suicide data can even be regarded as reliable. Despite possible shortcomings, Durkheim's study represents a major attempt to relate the individual and the wider society. In it, he identifies two dimensions for understanding the state of balance in society. The first involves the rules and moral norms that regulate social life and operate to curtail individual excesses, while the second concerns the ways in which individuals fit into and have a sense of belonging to society.

Durkheim believed that both social integration and social regulation con-tributed to rates of suicide, either by being insufficient or excessive. It was a matter of balance. It is the consequences of loss of social regulation – anomie – that we shall consider here.

To take just one of the examples he uses, following a financial crisis in 1873 the numbers of suicides in Vienna rose from 141 in 1872 to 216 two years later. Durkheim considers what he describes as a 'seductively simple' explanation: that the additional suicides resulted from the increased difficulties and poverty people faced. He rejects this, showing that suicide rates also rose during periods of prosperity. For instance, the unification of Italy (in 1871) laid the basis for a period of substantial economic growth, with accompanying increases in wages. Despite this, from 1871 to 1877 the suicide rate in Italy rose from 31 per million to 40.6 per million, an increase of 36 per cent.

Several other similar examples are employed by Durkheim to support his conclusion that: 'When society is disturbed by some painful crisis or by beneficent but abrupt transitions, it is momentarily incapable of exercising this influence; thence come the sudden rises in the curve of suicides' (Cited in Thompson and Tunstall 1971: 115).

As Craib has put it, anomic suicide occurs when: 'the rules that govern social life fail and we are left not knowing how to behave, or what is appropriate' (Craib 1997: 31).

Traditional rules lose their authority at the very point when individual desires need greatest restraint: 'Their very demands make fulfilment impossible. Overweening ambition always exceeds the results obtained ... Nothing gives satisfaction and all this agitation is uninterruptedly maintained without appeasement' (Cited in Thompson and Tunstall 1971: 116).

It was, therefore, not the material consequences of financial crises that were important but the disruptive impact they had upon the 'collective order':

> If therefore industrial or financial crises increase suicides, this is not because they cause poverty, since crises of prosperity have the same result; it is because they are crises, that is, disturbances of the collective order ... Whenever serious readjustments take place in the social order, whether or not due to a sudden growth or to an unexpected catastrophe, men are more inclined to self-destruction. How is this possible? How can something considered generally to improve existence serve to detach men from it?
>
> (Cited in Thompson and Tunstall 1971: 108–9)

Social norms and personal rewards

Durkheim devotes considerable attention to investigating the social restraints that operate on people as they pursue the resources required to lead a happy and secure life. Pointing out that the desires of individuals could be insatiable, Durkheim argues that it is only by moral force that these can be regulated and that 'society alone can play this moderating role; for it is the only moral power superior to the individual, the authority of which he accepts'.

Durkheim is suggesting that within society we develop a general consensus around the rewards to which people are entitled:

> According to accepted ideas, for example, a certain way of living is considered the upper limit to which a workman may aspire in his efforts to improve his

existence, and there is another limit below which he is not willingly permitted to fall unless he has seriously demeaned himself. Both differ for city and country workers, for the domestic servant and the day-labourer, for the business clerk and the official, etc. Likewise the man of wealth is reproved if he lives the life of a poor man, but also if he seeks the refinements of luxury overmuch. Economists may protest in vain; public feelings will always be scandalized if an individual spends too much wealth for wholly superfluous use, and it even seems that this severity relaxes only in times of moral disturbance. A genuine regimen exists, therefore, although not always legally formulated, which fixes with relative precision the maximum degree of ease of living to which each social class may legitimately aspire. However, there is nothing immutable about such a scale. It changes with the increase or decrease of collective revenue and the changes occurring in the moral ideas of society. Thus what appears luxury to one period no longer does so to another; and the well-being which for long periods was granted to a class only by exception and superogation finally appears strictly necessary and equitable.

(Cited in Thompson and Tunstall 1971: 112)

Durkheim's argument is that social norms develop around what different groups and occupations are entitled to receive, and these provide us with a sense of having a 'fair reward'. We may want to earn more but we accept that what we are paid reflects the social 'worth' placed on our job. Durkheim goes on to develop this point by adding that it is not only necessary for the 'justice of the hierarchy of functions' to be accepted, it is also important that we feel our place within this has been determined fairly. Durkheim was deeply interested in how people perceived the justice of social arrangements and their place within them.

This is the aspect of Durkheim's thought that provides a fruitful way of thinking about the association between inequalities in health and income that Wilkinson has observed. It has special relevance in the context of a society, such as in Britain, where inequalities in wealth have continued to widen. To use just one example, in 2003 the average pay of senior company directors rose by 12.8 per cent, three times more than average earnings. This followed a 23 per cent average rise in the previous year and 17 per cent in the year before that. Including benefits from share options, the average pay of a chief executive in these companies was £1.7 million. Average pay in Britain is £24,600 (Finch and Treanor 2004: 1).

Durkheim regarded inequality as a threat to people's willingness to accept social norms, similar to the disorientation he saw caused by major social upheaval. A sense that some groups in society receive excessive rewards may undermine an acceptance of norms that would otherwise sustain a degree of mutual 'self-denial'. Although this argument cannot be developed further here, a contemporary example of rapid social change provides a stark illustration of the impact the wider social environment can have upon health status.

Social change and mortality in Russia

Mortality rates in the former communist countries in the Soviet Union and Eastern Europe rose after the fall of communism in 1989 to such an extent that in the subsequent decade four million *more* deaths occurred than would have been expected had the previous historical trend continued. Although not quite on the same scale, the numbers involved bear comparison with an estimated nine million deaths during the horrific period of civil war, famine and malnutrition in the 1920s (Cornia and Pannicia 2000).

As we have seen, Durkheim regarded anomie, and its associated negative consequences for health, as a potential consequence of rapid social change. A similar interpretation has been made by an international group of researchers, from Sweden, Russian and the UK, examining recent Russian mortality trends in Russia (Walberg *et al.* 1998).

Life expectancy among the Russian people living in the former Soviet Union began to show a steady improvement following the Second World War, although lagged behind the West by the 1960s. A substantial improvement in the mid-1980s, associated with an intense campaign aimed at reducing alcohol consumption, was not maintained with the ending of the Soviet Union. Between 1990 and 1994 average life expectancy at birth fell by five years. Among men, in the quarter of regions showing the greatest reduction in life expectancy, there was a fall of 8.6 years. Forty per cent of the total decline in life expectancy among this group of men was attributable to deaths within the 40 to 54 age group.

Overall, the regions with the largest falls in life expectancy were mainly urban, having high rates of labour turnover, greater income inequalities and higher crime rates. The labour turnover was measured using data from large- and medium-sized enterprises on the net number of job gains and job losses as a percentage of average employment. This is intended as an indicator of 'transition' or 'labour market shock'.

The authors refer to Durkheim's work on anomic suicide, describing it as being 'extraordinarily prescient in the Russian context':

> For Durkheim, rapid change results in a temporary disruption of the normal mechanisms through which society imposes limits on behaviour, which in turn results in increased rates of suicide. Although the mortality crisis in Russia has effected many other causes of death in addition to suicide, Durkheim's emphasis on the negative consequences of rapid social and economic change fits well with what we have found with respect to the importance of pace of change in explaining regional variations in mortality trends in Russia.
>
> (Walberg *et al.* 1998: 317)

The authors also suggest that their findings may have wider relevance for understanding the relationship between dramatic social upheavals and individual health. For example, they note that:

although the scale of the transition in Russia is extreme, it is not unique and there is now considerable evidence that the groups most affected in Russia, particularly young men and men in early middle age, have also suffered from the effects of transition elsewhere. Such effects may also be detectable, albeit on a smaller scale, in other settings, such as parts of western Europe that are becoming de-industrialised. This would be consistent with the literature on the health effects of unemployment and fear of unemployment.

(Walberg *et al.* 1998: 317)

Health professionals may be no better positioned than any other citizen to influence the character of social and economic changes but are well placed to reflect on the consequences for individuals. Failure to do so can result in health care needs being misunderstood or unmet. This issue is discussed in Chapter 10, in relation to access to health services, but before this, the following chapter continues to focus on psychosocial aspects by considering the role of workplace-related factors.

9
Work, control and health

The workplace as a source of ill-health provides the focus for the first part of this chapter which begins by introducing some of the ideas of Karl Marx on the relationship between working hours and health. This is followed by a description of data from the Whitehall studies previously referred to, looking at factors associated with coronary heart disease in particular. An explanation of how Marx used the concept of alienation to understand work experiences provides an opportunity to consider the issue of control in the workplace, including claims that the jobs of many employees have become 'deskilled'.

The second part of the chapter remains with the theme of organizational factors in the workplace but focuses more directly on the context of health care. The psychosocial character of illness does not only involve factors that may cause it, but also the manner in which it is dealt. An objective in this discussion is to bring attention back to relationships between patients and professionals, this time placing them within their institutional context.

Marx and the 'work–life balance'

It has become popular in many circles to speak of a 'work–life balance', reflecting fears that the demands of paid employment exact too high a price in terms of personal and family relationships. In part this may be a consequence of working hours, with British workers working amongst the longest in Europe, but there are also concerns about intensified pressures on people while at work. This can make it difficult to 'switch off', as matters related to one's job intrude into everyday life, disrupting a more balanced equilibrium.

The phrase, 'work–life balance', may be relatively new but the concerns are long-standing. One person who wrote passionately about the damaging effects of longer working hours in the mid-nineteenth century was Karl Marx. Marx's writings are often presented in a way that focuses on 'macro' economic relationships and systems, with little apparent attention to the individual but this neglects some important and powerful writing. Examples of this are used below to illustrate his approach.

Some words that he uses may now be unfamiliar, and the constant assumption that a worker is male is unhelpful, but attention needs only to be given to the general tenor. One term requiring explanation is the phrase 'labour process'. This refers to the circumstances under which work is performed and within capitalism Marx regarded it as exhibiting two characteristic phenomena: 'First, the worker works under the control of the capitalist to whom his labour belongs ... Secondly, the product is the property of the capitalist and not that of the worker, its immediate producer' (Marx 1976: 291–2).

For Marx, these features set the context for the manner in which work is performed. Control over work and what it produces is exercised by the employer rather than the employee. This can be illustrated by turning to Marx's comments on the impact of the length of the working day. Summing up a preceding section of his book, *Capital*, Marx delivers a damning indictment of changes designed to raise the productivity of labour:

> We saw ... that within the capitalist system all methods for raising the social productivity of labour are put into effect at the cost of the individual worker; that all means for the development of production undergo a dialectical inversion so that they become means of domination and exploitation of the producers; they distort the worker into a fragment of a man; they degrade him to the level of an appendage of a machine, they destroy the actual content of his labour by turning it into a torment; they alienate from him the intellectual potentialities of the labour process in the same proportion as science is incorporated in it as an independent power; they deform the conditions under which he works, subject him during the labour process to a despotism the more hateful for its meanness; they transform his life-time into working-time, and drag his wife and child beneath the wheels of the juggernaut of capital.
>
> (Marx 1976: 798–9)

The more emollient language of 'work–life balance' represents a modern-day reflection of this argument. But a moderation of language and passion can sometimes be associated with a softening of critical analysis. Marx was certainly prepared to challenge the status quo but does his analysis retain any relevance today? Consider the following comments from Marx, based on a newspaper item from January 1866:

> In London three railwaymen – a guard, an engine-driver, and a signalman – are up before a coroner's jury. A tremendous railway accident has dispatched hundreds of passengers into the next world. The negligence of the railway workers is the cause of the misfortune. They declare with one voice before the jury that ten or twelve years before their labour lasted only 8 hours a day. During the last five or six years, they say, it is screwed up to 14, 18 and 20 hours, and when the pressure of holiday travellers is especially severe, when excursion trains are put on, their labour often lasts for 40 or 50 hours without a break. They are ordinary men, not Cyclops. At a certain point their labour-power ran out. Torpor seized them. Their brains stopped thinking, their eyes

stopped seeing. The thoroughly 'respectable British Juryman' replied with a verdict that sent them to the Assizes on a charge of manslaughter.

(Marx 1976: 363)

Marx on working hours and health

Example after example is used by Marx to demonstrate the damage done to people's health by long working hours. Many are drawn from surgeons, physicians and public health specialists, leading Marx to conclude that working excessive hours:

> usurps the time for growth, development and healthy maintenance of the body. It steals the time required for the consumption of fresh air and sunlight. It haggles over the meal-times, where possible incorporating them into the production process itself, so that food is added to the worker as to a mere means of production, as coal is supplied to the boiler, and grease and oil to the machinery. It reduces the sound sleep needed for the restoration, renewal and refreshment of the vital forces to the exact amount of torpor essential to the revival of an absolutely exhausted organism.
>
> (Marx 1976: 375–6)

While the phrase 'psychosocial' might have been unfamiliar to Marx, the essential concept was not. But Marx's purpose in describing the damaging effects of the lengthening working day was not simply to deliver a humanistic rebuke of its effects. His primary interest was in exploring the factors that would eventually regulate and limit working hours.

Tracing the statutory restrictions placed on child labour in 1833, 1844 and 1847, Marx deplores the success with which many employers evaded the laws. However, as rising labour protests prompted further legislation, the Factory Act of 1850 for the first time regulated the working day of all workers within defined industries. By the 1860s more industries were being brought within its purview. Although referring to it as a 'modest Magna Carta of the legally limited working day', Marx quotes a Factory Inspectors' Report, 'which at last makes clear "when the time which the workers sells is ended, and when his own begins"'. Quoting Virgil, Marx adds, 'What a great change from that time!'

Contemporary developments

For Marx, the main lesson of the movement for 'protection' is that: 'the workers have to put their heads together and, as a class, compel the passing of a law, an all-powerful social barrier by which they can be prevented from selling themselves and their families into slavery and death by voluntary contract with capital' (Marx 1976: 416).

Further changes were achieved, with an eight-hour working day being one of the central demands of many trade unions in the late nineteenth century. Improvements continued through much of the twentieth century but recent years have seen something of a reversal. In the spring of 2001, the average weekly hours worked by full-time employed males in the European Union was a little over 42, compared to almost 46 in the UK. The UK not only has the longest working hours, it also has far fewer statutory holidays. Perhaps more important is the distribution of the hours that is concealed by the overall averages:

> Although most full-time employees in the United Kingdom work 40 hours, the range of the distribution of usual working hours is wider. A quarter of full-time employees usually work 38 hours or less, but another quarter usually work 48 hours or over.
>
> (Van Bastelaer and Vaguer 2004)

According to a report produced in December 2002 by the recruitment company, Manpower, one in ten UK workers works at least 61 hours a week. In addition to long hours, workers in the UK are also more likely to work outside normal daytime hours on weekdays – here the proportion is one in three, compared with less than one in five in Luxembourg. Nor is this evenly distributed, with at least half of low-skilled, non-manual employees working outside these normal hours (Manpower 2002).

This is accompanied by an increasing amount of shift work, with the proportion of UK workers working shifts rising from 12 per cent in 1992 to 14 per cent in 1997 (Social Trends 1998). Traditionally used in continuous manufacturing processes, as well as many areas of human service work such as health and social care, shift work has become increasingly common in other sectors, such as retailing and leisure. The proportion working shifts in sales almost doubled during this five-year period.

Evidence of lengthening working hours with more use of shift work also comes from the data of children born in 1946, 1958 and 1970 (described in the previous chapter). On average, men born in 1946 reported working 47.2 hours a week in their early 30s, compared to an average of 44.6 hours by those born in 1958 at the same age. However, the average for the 1970 cohort at age 30 was 47.1 hours, effectively the same as for the 1946 cohort. (Ferri, Bynner and Wadsworth 2003)

While causal relationships are inevitably difficult to identify, it is noteworthy that the increasing number of hours being worked is accompanied by a small reduction in the proportion of parents stating that child care is equally shared between them. Members of cohorts from 1958 and 1970, and who were parents in their early 30s, were asked about their contribution to child care. This did not require any supporting evidence and was simply the individual's own judgement, however, quite high proportions of men and women in both cohorts described it as being shared equally. This was particularly so where either both or neither were in employment.

Sixty-one per cent of men and 53 per cent of women born in 1958 described child care as being shared equally, slightly higher than the proportions reported by the 1970 cohort (59 per cent and 46 per cent) (Ferri, Bynner and Wadsworth 2003). The decline may not be great but the fact that it is a decline rather than a continuing upward trend could suggest an influence of increasing working hours on personal and family relationships. Although these may appear outside of the direct ability of health professionals to control, history suggests that securing social constraints on these developments can be assisted by the contributions of health professionals, working in concert with other social movements.

The central issue is one of how problems are defined: and whose problem they are seen to be. It can be very easy to emphasize the responsibility of the individual to lead a healthy life while at the same time neglect powerful obstacles that may be placed in the way. Marx was appalled at the escalating working hours many workers were expected to perform and welcomed the legislative controls eventually imposed on them. He was incensed at the 'degradation', 'domination', 'despotism' and 'alienation' he saw as characterizing workplace relationships within capitalism. Marx wrote with feeling about the world around him and a central concern was that workers become components in a system of work organization over which they have little or no control. He uses the concept of alienation to explain this, a concept we will return to, after briefly reviewing some contemporary evidence on the possible relationship between health and control in the workplace.

Health and control in the workplace

Important data in this area has been generated by studies of coronary heart disease among London-based civil servants, often referred to as the Whitehall and Whitehall II studies. The Whitehall II study involved a sample drawn from a population of all London-based civil service office staff aged 35–55. The final cohort was made up of 10,308 staff, mostly white-collar but ranging from office support to permanent secretary. Between 1985 and 1988 baseline information was collected on a range of individual health details, including data on height, weight, blood pressure, serum cholesterol, lifestyle, work characteristics, social support and significant life events. A series of subsequent questionnaires and screenings took place, up to the period 1997–9. By this time, three-quarters of those who had originally volunteered were still participating.

The results showed steep gradients in health status from the lower to higher occupational groups, which were maintained throughout the 11 years of the study. Generally the differences in health status between occupational groups remained fairly constant, however, the study also looked at levels of depression, for which this was not the case. Measured using the General Health Questionnaire score, inequalities in the distribution of depression across occupational groups widened during the period (Ferrie et al. 2002). This appears to have been the result of considerable improvements in the higher grades and deterioration in the lower grades. Several possible explanations for these trends are considered in the study, with the authors concluding: 'Of these explanations the deteriorating working conditions and the increased likelihood of physical illness in the lower grades seem the most plausible and demand further analysis in the future' (Ferrie et al. 2002).

Drawing on the results of the Whitehall studies, Michael Marmot comments on the complexity of processes involved. For example, low-grade posts may involve lower levels of job control but a higher proportion of those who hold them smoke and do less exercise. Nevertheless, analysis to control for these different factors continues to lead to the conclusion: 'Statistically, low control makes a substantial independent contribution to the social gradient in heart disease' (Marmot 2004: 130).

The studies also identified statistically different rates between occupational groups for minor psychiatric disorders. 'Minor' disorders, distinguished from 'major' disorders such as schizophrenia and manic depression, include anxiety and depression, conditions which contribute to substantial levels of certified sickness. Ninety-one million working days are lost each year due to mental health problems, half of which are attributable to anxiety and stress conditions (Gray 1999: 2).

Workplace experiences do not arise in isolation from other aspects of our lives and Marmot points to a need to take account of this wider context, including home circumstances:

> The lower the level of control over work, the greater is the risk of developing minor psychiatric disorder. Low control was a major part of the explanation of the social gradient in depressive symptoms . . .
>
> We found that people who reported low control at home had a higher risk of depression. This risk was in addition to the risk of depression associated with low control at work. Particularly striking was the high risk of depression in low-status women who told us they had little control over things at home. Our interpretation was that for these low-status women, work offers little in the way of psychological reward.
>
> (Marmot 2004: 130–2)

Turning to the results on coronary heart disease, one of the research papers published as part of the Whitehall II study, concludes:

> Men and women with low job control, either self reported or independently assessed, had a higher risk of newly reported coronary heart disease during follow up . . . The cumulative effect of low job control assessed on two occasions indicates that giving employees more variety in tasks and a stronger say in decisions about work may decrease the risk of coronary heart disease.
>
> (Bosma et al. 1997: 558)

Similarly, a review of research literature on the association between conditions and relationships at work and psychological and physical ill-health (focusing on the specific experiences of women) observes:

> The degree of power which other people have over the conduct of an individual's working day – 'work control' – has been shown to be central in this relationship. The effect of control at work does not seem, in these studies, to be produced by different lifestyles, in terms of diet, leisure exercise or smoking. Rather, the effect may be produced by a bio-psychosocial process in

which stress caused by low control and monotony at work induces changes both in mood and in blood chemistry.

(Brunner 1997)

One further example, drawn from Finland, comes from a study that sought to explore the dynamics involved by examining the effects of 'job-strain' and 'effort–reward imbalance'. 'Job strain' describes situations where high work demands combine with low levels of job control; while 'effort–reward' imbalance refers to factors such as earnings, job security and career, which may be affected by wider labour market factors and not merely the effort actually expended. The study was conducted in a factory in Finland, examining rates of cardiovascular mortality between 1973 and 2001. Questionnaires were used to gain information about the two key topics, each of which has been suggested to be a source of adverse consequences for health.

Eight hundred and twelve employees were selected, representative of the whole workforce in terms of sex, age and occupational group, none of whom showed evidence of cardiovascular disease in 1973. During the following 28 years, 73 of the original sample died of cardiovascular disease. Various demographic, behavioural and biological factors were found to be associated with these deaths. The authors of the study note: 'As expected, higher age, male sex, low worker status, smoking, sedentary lifestyle, high blood pressure, high cholesterol concentration, and high body mass index increased the risk of death' (Kivimaki et al. 2002: 858).

For example, smokers were more than twice as likely to have died as non-smokers and those who had low levels of physical activity were around two and a half times more likely to die as those with high levels of activity. As the authors indicate, none of this is surprising, confirming the relationship between these factors and cardiovascular disease. But beyond these behavioural and lifestyle influences, other factors could have just as much impact: 'Employees scoring high on job strain and effort-reward imbalance had a twofold risk of death compared with their colleagues with low strain and low effort-reward imbalance.'

The data also revealed: 'At follow up, concentrations of total cholesterol increased for employees with high job strain and low job control, and body mass index increased for employees with low job control and high effort–reward imbalance' (Kivimaki et al. 2002: 858).

However, the precise impact of low job control on mortality seemed to vary between occupational groups, having greater effect on those with lower status occupations. Similar results were found in a separate study by Lynch et al. (1997).

Marx: work control and alienation

Having illustrated the growing empirical evidence on the association between work control and health, we can return to the work of Karl Marx, particularly to his use of the concept of alienation. The concept is difficult to define in a way that provides a measurable category for use in empirical research, but it, nevertheless, has value in helping us think about the character of social relationships in the workplace.

Marx's objections to the increasing hours many workers were required to work have been noted. He was equally concerned about the conditions in which labour was performed, not simply the physical conditions but the social relationships between worker and employer. It was in this context that he uses the concept of alienation, described in one of his earlier works in the following way:

> In what does this alienation of labour consist? First, that the work is external to the worker, that it is not a part of his nature, that consequently he does not fulfil himself in his work but denies himself, has a feeling of misery, not of well-being, does not develop freely a physical and mental energy, but is physically exhausted and mentally debased. The worker therefore feels himself at home only during his leisure, whereas at work he feels homeless. His work is not voluntary but imposed, forced labour. It is not the satisfaction of a need, but only a means for satisfying other needs. Its alien character is clearly shown by the fact that as soon as there is no physical or other compulsion it is avoided like the plague.
>
> (Cited in Bottomore and Rubel 1963: 177–8)

Marx has been criticized for adopting an impossibly optimistic view of how work might be organized differently. Remarks he wrote in *The German Ideology* are sometimes held up for ridicule, where he offers an image of the future society:

> where nobody has one exclusive sphere of activity but each can become accomplished in any branch he wishes, society regulates the general production and thus makes it possible for me to do one thing today and another tomorrow, to hunt in the morning, fish in the afternoon, rear cattle in the evening, criticize after dinner, just as I have a mind, without ever becoming hunter, fisherman, shepherd or critic.

Francis Wheen, commenting that this somewhat exhausting Nirvana does not indicate who will clean the lavatories or hew the coal, also notes that Marx later described *The German Ideology* as having been primarily a stimulus to thinking: 'We abandoned the manuscript to the gnawing of the mice, all the more willingly as we had achieved our main purpose – self-clarification' (Quoted in Wheen 1999: 97).

This did not mean he abandoned the underlying concept. Marx's thinking about alienation was influenced by the philosopher Ludwig Feurbach, who used the expression to describe: 'a condition in which man's own powers appeared as self-subsistent forces or entities controlling his actions' (Bottomore and Rubel 1963: 20).

Feurbach employs the concept of alienation in an account of religion, arguing that humans project themselves into the image of a God, an image that then becomes reified, that is, made more real and concrete. Laws which, in reality, originate with people, come to be regarded as divine laws. They are alien in the sense of being regarded as external, beyond human control.

Marx retains a parallel meaning to Feurbach's use of the concept of alienation. It is not simply boredom or frustration but a sense that the product of our work, and the work itself, appear as alien, as external and beyond our control. For Marx there were several dimensions to such alienation but one involved a tendency towards labour itself becoming alienating, as labour is transformed into a commodity like any other. This, he believed, causes it to lose any real meaning, as it no longer forms part of our own sense of being. The labour being performed comes to be seen as something 'external' to the worker. Marx goes on to consider what it is that creates such alienating conditions:

> If the product of labour does not belong to the worker, if it confronts him as an alien power, this can only be because it belongs to some other man than the worker ... If his own activity is to him an unfree activity, then he is treating it as activity performed in the service, under the dominion, the coercion and the yoke of another man.
>
> (Cited in Burns 1969: 105)

Taylorism and the 'deskilling thesis'

For many years, Marx's writings on work and alienation were comparatively neglected. Some saw them as representative of his humanistic, youthful output, from which the more 'mature' Marx moved on to focus on economic analysis. However, Marx's writings on the labour process received renewed attention with the publication of *Labor and Monopoly Capital*, in 1974. Written by Harry Braverman, the book sought to apply Karl Marx's analysis of the control of labour to American employment in the twentieth century. For a time his book was very influential, even though many have challenged important elements of the historical account.

The ensuing arguments over historical interpretation need not concern us, but a highly important contribution of Braverman was to direct attention to processes in the workplace he described as 'deskilling':

> The concept of deskilling refers to four processes: (i) the process whereby the shopfloor loses the right to design and plan work; i.e. divorce of planning and doing; (ii) the fragmentation of work into meaningless segments; (iii) the redistribution of tasks amongst unskilled and semi-skilled labour, associated with labour cheapening; and (iv) the transformation of work organization from the craft system to modern, Taylorized forms of labour control.
>
> (Littler 1982: 25)

'Taylorism' refers to a body of thinking, described by its founder, Frederick Taylor, as 'scientific management'. Taylor's book, *Principles of Scientific Management*, was published in 1911 and although these principles were probably not as widely adopted as Braverman tends to assume, they provide a helpful summation of a particular model of management. Fundamental to this is the issue of control:

> The work of every workman is fully planned out by the management at least one day in advance, and each man received in most cases complete written

instructions, describing in detail the task which he is to accomplish, as well as
the means to be used in doing the work ... This task specifies not only what is
to be done but how it is to be done and the exact time allowed for it.

(Taylor 1911: 39)

Taylor believed that organizing work in this way would increase efficiency,
removing from the worker any need to think or make decisions about what actions
to take. By describing and prescribing each element of work, every moment of the
working day could be used productively. Associated with this, Taylor believed the
number of tasks performed by each individual at all levels in an organization
should be as few as possible:

Functional management consists in so dividing the work of management that
each man from the assistant superintendent down shall have as few functions
as possible to perform. If practicable the work of each man in the management
should be confined to the performance of a single leading function.

(Taylor 1911: 99)

There is much else in Taylor's model of management but the underlying idea
was that management was a science, and its main objective was to separate out the
individual tasks that constituted a work process, organizing the performance of
them in such a way as to achieve maximum efficiency. Images of mass production
lines exemplify this, epitomized in the Charlie Chaplin film, 'Modern Times'.

Braverman argued that employment in the twentieth century was increasingly
dominated by the application of Taylorist principles, resulting in the deskilling of
workers, unable to exercise control over the method or pace of their work. This
contention stimulated a long-running controversy, the 'deskilling debate', with
many arguing that Braverman's interpretation was one-dimensional, offering a
superficial view of the concept of 'skill'. This debate cannot be adequately summarized here and it should be acknowledged that a considerable number of jobs do
not fit Braverman's description. But many do. At the very least, Braverman's
deskilling thesis offers a way of thinking about the factors that contribute to a lack
of control at work.

Health, work and unemployment

Reference must also be made to another aspect of the relationship between health
and work. This concerns not the intensification or control of work, but its absence.
Wilkinson identifies studies of unemployment as providing some of the 'clearest
indications that relative deprivation affects health through psychosocial channels'
(Wilkinson 1996: 177).

Referring to early research questions about whether unemployment caused
poor health, or if ill people are more likely to become unemployed, he notes the
results of studies into factory closures that demonstrate a deterioration in health as
a consequence of unemployment:

But, even more interesting, these same studies also showed that much of the deterioration in health started, not when people actually became unemployed, but before that – when redundancies were first announced. It now turns out that a large part of the link between health and unemployment is related to job insecurity and the anticipation of unemployment ... It provides powerful evidence that one of the clearest categories of deprivation in modern societies affects health predominantly through psychosocial channels.

(Wilkinson 1992: 178)

Problems arising from the social distribution of work, with too much for some and too little for others, were noted three-quarters of a century ago by the philosopher, Bertrand Russell. In an essay written in 1935, 'In Praise of Idleness', Russell observed:

Modern methods of production have given us the possibility of ease and security for all; we have chosen instead, to have overwork for some and starvation for the others. Hitherto we have continued to be as energetic as we were before there were machines; in this we have been foolish, but there is no reason to go on being foolish for ever.

(Russell 1976: 25)

Much of what has happened in the 70 years since that was written seems to suggest otherwise. However, it should not be assumed people are powerless to resist changes within the workplace.

Control and resistance

Marx, as we have seen, saw collective action by the emerging labour movement as the basis for opposition. In his own lifetime, trade union membership was largely restricted to skilled workers but by the end of the nineteenth century this was starting to change. 'New unionism' extended collective organization to the ranks of semi-skilled and unskilled workers and between 1910 and 1920 the proportion of British workers who were members of trade unions rose from just 16 per cent to 48 per cent (Bain and Price 1983).

Substantial membership losses occurred during the 1920s and 1930s but during the years after World War Two the upward rise returned. The peak was reached in 1979, when there were 12.7 million members, representing nearly 54 per cent of the workforce. Since then, membership has tumbled to 7.3 million, 29 per cent of employees (Palmer, Granger and Fitzner 2004).

Nevertheless, with more than seven million members, unions retain a significant role. They continue to provide an important channel for representing workplace grievances and a vehicle by which employees can seek to resist unreasonable demands. However, the decline in trade union membership has been accompanied by its concentration in a limited number of employment sectors. Changes in the economy and the labour market have meant there are now many areas of employment where membership is minimal.

Despite this decline, efforts to retain a measure of control are still likely to be made. They may simply take a more individual form. Examples of this can be found in a study that interviewed a group of Glasgow men, aged between 30 and 49, about the relationship between health and work (Mullen 1992). Methods used were qualitative ones, unlike the use of quantitative data in the large-scale Whitehall surveys. The aim was to explore experiences and attitudes, and how health was understood.

In the interviews, health was often related to experiences of work. This could be in both positive and negative ways. One issue concerned how people dealt with situations where the pressures from work became too much, described in the study as 'compensation strategies':

> interviewees highlighted forms of disengagement where they could consciously distance themselves from involvement in the work process. This took the form of either physical or mental disengagement. Such disengagement can be seen as a form of role-distance. When, for one reason or another, the given time structure of work became too oppressive, respondents often cut themselves off from a too close involvement with their work duties. Such disengagement may be physical and involve leaving the immediate workspace, going to another department of their factory or office ... Mental disengagement, by contrast, involved some form of role-distance, not allowing oneself to become too involved with one's task. Again, which respondents could utilise which form of disengagement depended on the degrees of control they had over the structuring of their work tasks and also the extent to which they were supervised.

> Time disengagement, be it physical or mental, was closely related to feelings of stress and their relief. Indeed respondents stated that they had changed their approach to work when they had gone through a period of crisis or if they had seen a colleague go through such a period. One respondent described his changing attitude to work after suffering the symptoms of a heart attack. He said now 'work can wait'.

> (Mullen 1992: 80–1)

This would have horrified Frederick Taylor, and many employers (and possibly work colleagues) are likely to discourage such behaviour. But it can be seen as an individual response to pressures of work that might otherwise be damaging. 'Taking a sickie' may sometimes have positive benefits for the longer term. Without a reasonable and sustainable equilibrium between different aspects of life, far too many people can be at risk of being dragged 'beneath the wheels of the juggernaut of capital'.

Marx's other message is that achieving a balance between 'work' and 'life', as if they form two distinct categories, is not sufficient. Reasserting control over the hours of work individuals perform is important but so too is a recognition that the work itself should be satisfying. Although there may be limits to what can be done directly by health professionals in these areas, there is a potential for these issues to be given much greater prominence as public health issues. Defining the problem of coronary heart disease as one that puts responsibilities on employing organizations as well as on individuals could represent an important shift in how modern patterns of illness are understood.

The remainder of this chapter considers another way in which the literature and research evidence in this area might be applied to organizational relationships within health care. Attention has already been given to relationships between a patient and a health care professional, but these do not exist in isolation. In many ways, they reflect the contours of the broader institutional arrangements within which they are established.

Health care, hierarchies and control

The inquiry into events at the Bristol Royal Infirmary addressed not only the interactions between patients, parents and professionals, it also explored wider relationships within the NHS. One observation, drawing attention to the relationship between 'old-style paternalism' and hierarchy, is particularly worth noting:

> The continued existence of a hierarchical approach within and between the healthcare professions is a significant cultural weakness. While the situation has changed somewhat over the past decade or so, the problem remains. Even today, in some places, it is assumed that a doctor's view is inevitably superior and that nurses are there to carry out a doctor's orders. This continues despite the very great efforts made by the nursing profession to create a relationship of mutual dependence and respect between doctors and nurses. Many nurses in hospitals and elsewhere still do not feel valued by their medical colleagues or by managers . . .
>
> (Kennedy 2001: 18)

> Subservience or deference to a perceived superior can be a particular barrier when issues arise among healthcare professionals about a colleague's performance. Although there is now a duty on doctors and nurses to protect patients from risk and not to suppress concerns about a colleague's performance, very many in practice today were educated and trained in a culture in which there was a reluctance to criticise or comment upon the conduct of colleagues, particularly those who were more senior or practised in the same team or specialty. This is the negative side of the tradition of group loyalty which has been a strength in times of relative adversity. It continues to be a negative aspect of NHS culture. Not only does it make it difficult for an individual to summon up the courage not to conform, but this sense of hierarchy also influences who gets listened to within the organisation when questions are raised.
>
> (Kennedy 2001: 19)

That report was published in 2001, a year after the Government had announced, in its NHS Plan, a far more optimistic future:

> Throughout the NHS the old hierarchical ways of working are giving way to more flexible team working between different clinical professionals. (para 9.2)
>
> The new approach will shatter the old demarcations which have held back staff and slowed down care. NHS employers will be required to empower appropriately qualified nurses, midwives and therapists to undertake a wider range of clinical tasks.
>
> (Secretary of State for Health 2000: para 9.5)

In fact, the focus of this statement is not so much upon hierarchical relationships, as upon interprofessional relationships. One way of thinking of this is in terms of hierarchical relationships existing on a vertical dimension, from top to bottom, and interprofessional relationships on a horizontal dimension. The two can combine, as with the kind of hierarchical distinctions between professions criticized by the Bristol Inquiry report. Challenging demarcation boundaries between professions may require a challenge to hierarchical power structures, but this need not be the case.

Technocratic challenges to professional authority

The principle of 'professional autonomy' represented one of the founding principles of the NHS (Allsop 1995). The idea was that professionals were best placed to make decisions about care and service provision, and should do so with administrative support rather than managerial intervention. In reality, this generally applied only to the medical profession but by the 1960s some early indications were emerging that this notion was being challenged. In part coming from a consumerist direction, probably more significant was what has been described as the 'politics of technocratic change' and an 'ideology of efficiency' (Klein 1989). This was an approach incorporated into a substantial reorganization of the NHS in the 1970s.

The word 'managerialism' has been used to characterize this development, standing in contrast to an organizational model based on professional autonomy and control (see, for example, Haywood and Alaszewski 1980). It does not assume that professionalism represents the best safeguard for ensuring effective and efficient services. Concerns about efficiency came increasingly to the fore and by the early 1980s prompted the Prime Minister, Margaret Thatcher, to invite Roy Griffiths, of the supermarket chain Sainsbury, to propose new management arrangements for the NHS. Issues identified in his subsequent report included concern that professionals could obstruct change and that there was an apparent lack of anyone in charge of the NHS at local and hospital level. This perception led to the recommendation, swiftly implemented, to introduce 'general managers' into the NHS.

In a study of the impact of general management on nursing, Owens and Glennester concluded, however, that the 'structural changes were more apparent than real, as they did not signify changed power relationships' (Owens and Glennester 1990: 111).

Similarly, writing of the prospects facing health professions, Jan Salvage suggests change was not as extensive as might have been thought: 'Relationships between medicine and patients, other professionals and the state changed relatively little in the decades after 1948' (Salvage 2002: 6).

Referring to the conclusions of writers such as Owens and Glennester, other researchers drew different conclusions: 'With the hindsight of almost a decade we suggest that their scepticism is misplaced, and that the significance of the introduction of general management into the NHS lay in providing a structural basis for the introduction of an internal market and a reinvigorated form of Taylorism' (Walby et al. 1994: 134).

Both assessments may be relevant for understanding developments, perhaps pointing to contrasting consequences that emerged for different professional groups. It was one thing to subject professions such as nursing to new systems of workload assessment, but another to apply this to the medical profession.

Despite attempts by the state to 'chip away' at medical dominance, including attempts to bring it under tighter control with the introduction of general management, Salvage sees little evidence of success. One consequence, she believes, is that the work of nurses and other health professionals remains largely determined by a medically dominated system: 'Significantly, the settings and specialities where nurses began to develop more autonomous roles or innovations were those in which medicine had little stake, or where it had a vested interest in nurse empowerment' (Salvage 2002: 7).

These included the nurse practitioner role in the US, developed as a way of providing primary health care in inner-city or rural areas where doctors did not want to work. Similarly, the use of nurse practitioners and clinical nurse specialists in the UK has largely been driven by the pressures created by the reduction in junior doctors' hours:

> From the 1970s onwards nurses have been advancing new types of initiatives (characterised by a holistic approach involving the patient's active participation) covering many innovations in various settings, such as prescribing, clinical specialist practice, nurse consultations in primary health care, community empowerment, and projects with socially excluded groups. Yet managers and policy-makers mostly gave only lukewarm support until pragmatism forced them to adopt 'new' solutions.
>
> (Salvage 2002: 7)

Salvage alleges that change can be obstructed when it faces powerful opposition. Examples cited include the slow progress achieved in the introduction of nurse prescribing and the closure of the Oxford Nurse Development Unit. Nurses in this unit provided intermediate care for patients no longer requiring more intensive, medically-oriented care and treatment, and Salvage refers to studies that indicated it improved outcomes for patients, with fewer deaths and greater independence on discharge. Despite this, she claims the unit was forced to close because: 'research evidence could not override the opposition of some medical consultants who regarded it as an affront to their power' (Salvage 2002: 7).

Changing professional roles

In her paper, Salvage raises the question of whether the dominance of the doctor in the NHS is still appropriate. She urges a reconsideration of the GP's traditional 'gatekeeper' role, as almost the sole point of referral to specialists (an optician cannot refer a patient directly to an ophthalmologist, for example). Salvage's argument is that the attitudes and relationships in which traditional models of professionalism originated are no longer dominant in society:

> Partly springing from these broad societal changes, the demands, expectations and attitudes of patients are also shifting ... As the expert patient/carer becomes a common phenomenon, the professional's role needs to shift. The status of professionals of all types is changing from being the guardians of knowledge to being counsellors and interpreters (Handy 1998). Building relationships with patients and communities and empowering them whenever possible to manage their own health and illness, while continuing to care for those who are unable to help themselves, are at the core of the new professionalism.

> The rise of consumerism and the empowered patient, and the social transformations wrought by changing attitudes to gender, class and ethnicity, mean that society is less and less willing to give the professions free rein to conduct their own affairs. This is particularly clear following a string of highly publicised failures by the regulatory bodies to root out or punish malpractice. The traditional contract between professions and laity, with its specific rights and obligations, is wearing thin and professionals are increasingly seen as workers like any other.

> (Salvage 2002: 12)

The idea of reconsidering the GP gatekeeper role has already progressed to a limited extent with the establishment of nine pilot sites by the National Institute for Learning, Skills and Innovation (formerly the NHSU) as part of its First Contact programme: The first contact clinician is an experienced professional, specifically trained and accredited to be able to assess, diagnose and treat patients with undifferentiated diagnoses, taking on some of the work previously done by GPs' (Laird 2004: 42).

The former NHSU described the programme as helping appropriately qualified and experienced non-medical staff to:

> assess and diagnose patients accurately. You can then plan their treatment, refer them on to the most appropriate professional, advise them on self-care or discharge them as appropriate. It will help you work more efficiently as part of a team, and respond more effectively to patient needs. You'll also be gaining skills that are transferable within the NHS.

> For patients, the programme will mean greater choice and easier access to services. It will also reduce the length of time they have to wait before seeing a healthcare professional, and reduce the need for them to see a range of

different people. Ensuring that all patients see a primary care professional within 24 hours and a GP within 48 hours is a key goal in the NHS 10-year plan.

First Contact Care also supports the Changing Workforce Programme and the strategy for nursing, midwifery and health visiting, Making a Difference.

(NHSU website)

Opening up the potential for significant change, it is also appropriate to reflect on Salvage's suggestion that change can be driven by resource factors rather than a desire for innovation. Is this likely to genuinely improve the status and power of patients? Is it accurate to interpret current changes as representing challenges to existing hierarchical systems of control; or little more than a means of increasing the productivity of labour?

Problems of bureaucratic organization

From its inception, in 1948, the NHS was a hierarchical organization, a feature that remained through several substantial organizational changes. Allsop has described changes implemented following the 1989 'Working for Patients' White Paper in the following terms: 'The reforms ... signified a shift from the command and control economy to a managed model' (Allsop 1995).

That model still retained a fundamentally hierarchical structure. The introduction of general management in the 1980s frequently encouraged a structure based around vertically managed clinical directorates rather than on coordination across them. Systems of this kind possess many shortcomings but of particular importance in the context of health work is the relationship between hierarchical control and a work activity that is often unpredictable.

Although much is often said about reducing hierarchy and centralism in the NHS, the reality has been a plethora of centrally-driven targets, strategies, performance indicators and protocols. What might be the effects of this? The influence of formal systems and procedures upon employee behaviour has long attracted attention. Robert Merton, an American sociologist writing in 1940, suggested that 'bureaucratic organization' may have unintended consequences. Although the word bureaucracy has come to be associated with images of unnecessary officialdom and excessive administrative regulation, or 'red tape', it originated simply as a way of referring to formal, administrative processes. However, warned Merton:

> Rules, designed as means to ends, may well become ends in themselves ... Governed by similar work conditions officials develop a group solidarity which may result in opposition to necessary change. Where officials are supposed to serve the public the very norms of impersonality which govern their behaviour may cause conflict with individual citizens.

(Cited in Albrow 1970: 55)

Staff may stick to the letter rather than the spirit of the rules, giving rise to the sort of criticism that has been levelled at several public services in the past, of being unresponsive and lacking a 'customer focus'. In one study, the impact of ward routines was commented on by a hospital ward sister: 'We're having to think of our routines before our patient. But then, what is this hospital system? This is what happens. We've got to have a routine' (Hospital ward sister, quoted in James 1992).

An example of this can be seen in the delay in implementing early recommendations on relaxing visiting restrictions on children's wards. These were recommended in 1959 in the Platt Report but it became apparent that many hospitals retained very restrictive times for visiting. A subsequent investigation into why this occurred concluded that although the original inquiry had taken account of psychological aspects, little attention was given to sociological factors: 'Specifically, it appeared that the social implications for hospital organization had been insufficiently recognized' (Stacey *et al.* 1970: 4).

Another writer on these issues has pointed to the capacity for front-line workers to establish ways of working for themselves. Staff adopting this role are described as 'street-level bureaucrats'. This is seen as a response to conflicting objectives and limited resources, combined with a capacity to exercise a reasonably high level of discretion in carrying out their work: 'the decisions of street-level bureaucrats, the routines they establish and the devices they invent to cope with uncertainties and work pressures effectively *become* the policies they carry out' (Lipsky 1980: xii).

This can involve, suggests Lipsky, the adoption of strategies in which staff: 'modify their concept of their jobs, so as to lower or otherwise restrict their objectives and thus reduce the gap between available resources and achieving objectives' (Lipsky 1980: 82).

Markets and networks

Responses of this kind can be viewed as reactions to tensions created by an unwieldy bureaucratic system. However, these systems were already coming under pressure from other directions. The introduction of the 'internal market' in the early 1990s can be interpreted, to some extent, as a reaction against the shortcomings of bureaucratic systems. The term 'internal market' refers to the element of competition between 'self-governing trusts' that came with a separation of purchasing and provider roles in the NHS.

More recently, interest has been shown in the role of networks and team working. As a review of health care organizational systems across the world, conducted by the World Health Organization, observed: 'Both hierarchical bureaucracies and fragmented, unregulated markets have serious flaws as ways to organize services: flexible integration of autonomous or semi-autonomous health care providers can mitigate the problem' (World Health Organization 2000).

Similar changes have been observed in many organizational contexts. Examining developments in control arrangements more generally, the social theorist Manuel Castells, has suggested:

What emerges from the observation of major organizational change in the last two decades of the century is not a new, 'one best way' of production, but the crisis of an old, powerful but excessively rigid model associated with the large, vertical corporation, and with oligopolistic control over markets . . .

. . . recent historical experience has already provided some of the answers concerning the new organizational forms of the informational economy. Under different organizational arrangements, and through diverse expressions, they are all based in networks. Networks are the fundamental stuff of which new organizations are and will be made.

(Castells 1996: 167–8)

In the UK, one of the earliest examples of such an approach came in proposals to establish networks of cancer care services across England and Wales (Calman and Hine 1995). This prompted growing interest in what came to be described as 'managed clinical networks'. These were defined in a review of acute services in Scotland, recommending their introduction, as:

Linked groups of health professionals and organisations from primary, secondary and tertiary care, working in a coordinated manner, unconstrained by existing professional and health board boundaries to ensure equitable provision of high quality and clinically effective services throughout Scotland.

(The Scottish Office/Department of Health 1998)

The use of this approach in the US is noted in a paper on managed clinical networks produced by the former NHS South East Regional Office, which suggests:

the driver for integrated comprehensive healthcare systems in the United States is the realisation that the range of needs for humans is infinite and continuous, in comparison to the capability of traditional organisations to treat need which is finite and discontinuous. Integrated service provision, therefore, becomes the only way to match service and customer needs.

(SE Regional Office Working Group 2000: 4)

Team working

Much of this sounds positive and several very successful initiatives of this kind have been reported. One study that examined lessons from new forms of team working identified at least six important benefits that it could produce. These were: achieving better quality through coordination and collaboration; enabling joint initiatives; facilitating better care plans; producing more holistic care; achieving higher productivity and better use of resources; and increasing staff satisfaction (Opie 1997).

However, the development of effective team working is not without its problems, and the same study suggested seven specific potential difficulties:

inadequate organizational support; an absence of training; a lack of interprofessional trust; tensions between disciplines; imbalances of power; a marginalization of clients; and discontinuity of team membership.

None of these problems may be irresolvable but Opie makes the point that clarity around the purpose of the team work is essential:

> The objective of such teams – to achieve co-ordinated work is problematic. Does 'co-ordination' refer primarily to the co-ordination of administrative issues? i.e. the team knows that this person is to be discharged and will ensure that they have carried out their contribution to that discharge by the requisite date? Or does it mean bringing together knowledge from different professionals and from clients … setting in train a more complex process?
>
> (Opie 1997: 275)

The first could probably be achieved within existing hierarchical relationships between professional groups. Likely to improve administrative efficiency and contribute to a more effective use of resources, this may be welcomed. But will this substantially alter the experience of care? Possibly, in avoiding unnecessary delays, for instance; but political pressures to avoid 'bed blocking' derive, primarily, not from concerns about the welfare of an individual patient but from a desire to maximize use of the bed. Changes of this type do not imply a more fundamental reappraisal of existing authority relationships.

Challenges to these may prove controversial, as suggested in Jane Salvage's remarks on the demise of the Oxford Nurse Development Unit, but potential benefits also need to be considered. A contribution on this comes in a now rather dated study from the US (Simpson 1985). The research was conducted in four acute hospitals in San Fransisco, using questionnaires to measure the levels of responsibility and authority that nursing staff perceived themselves possessing. Other questionnaires were used to measure levels of job satisfaction, rates of staff turnover and absenteeism. These three dimensions were assumed to relate to the quality of patient care.

The results showed, perhaps unsurprisingly, that levels of perceived responsibility and authority were greatest at the level of director of nursing, at the top of the occupational hierarchy, and decreased towards the level of staff nurse. Of greater interest is a comparison of results between hospitals. This indicated that: 'the hospital whose staff nurses perceived lower authority scores also reported higher staff turnover, higher absenteeism rates and lower job satisfaction scores' (Simpson 1985: 347).

The two hospitals with the lowest job satisfaction scores had twice the rate of staff turnover and a considerably higher absenteeism rate than the two hospitals having the highest job satisfaction scores. Simpson concludes: 'It would seem that hospitals with low job satisfaction scores, high turnover and high absenteeism will not resolve this problem until they give autonomy to the staff nurses and allow them to utilize their knowledge base' (Simpson 1985: 347).

As earlier examples have demonstrated, low levels of employee control in the workplace contribute to poor health. Another consequence may be higher levels of absenteeism and staff turnover, contributing to a reduction in the quality of work. It may be that research into the relationship between health and control raises specific issues relevant to settings in which work is with people rather than objects. Challenges to power relationships embodied in traditional patient–professional relationships need to be accompanied by a simultaneous critique of the power relationships within which health care is organized.

This is particularly necessary in the context of the twin inequalities that have provided important strands running through this book: those associated with the patient–professional relationship and those relating to the social distribution of health. It is at this point that the two themes can be more directly connected, by addressing the question of whether the NHS achieves its historic objective of ensuring equality of access to health care.

10
Inequality and access to health care

The aim of this chapter is to link earlier themes relating to interaction and communication between professionals and patients, and those concerning social inequalities in health. One point needs to be stressed at the outset. Inequality is not being used as an alternative word for difference. Patients may differ, and receive different services, for a whole manner of reasons that are not indicative of an inequitable provision.

The historian, R.H. Tawney, challenges claims that reductions in inequalities require a simultaneous erosion of individual differences: 'While natural endowments differ profoundly, it is the mark of a civilized society to aim at eliminating such inequalities as have their source, not in individual differences but in its own organisation.' He goes on to add that genuine individuality is more likely to flourish in conditions that prevent unwarranted inequalities: 'Individual differences which are the source of social energy (are) more likely to ripen and find expression if social inequalities are, as far as practicable, diminished' (Tawney 1952: 49).

It is also necessary to avoid assumptions that attribute different outcomes simply to the effects of contrasting personal choices. Of course these may play a part but individual choice must be understood within the context in which it is made. This includes the range of information and alternatives that are available. In reality, a variety of factors influence how personal choices are made.

The inverse-care law

An important contribution to debates on the use of health care came in the early 1970s in a paper published in *The Lancet*. This suggested the existence of an 'inverse care law', whereby those with the most severe clinical needs can experience the greatest difficulty accessing services. The author, Julian Tudor Hart, was a GP working in a South Wales mining community, having moved from general practice in a relatively affluent area in London. He had been struck by the contrast in provision between the two areas, leading him to argue:

> In areas with most sickness and death, general practitioners have more work, larger lists, less hospital support and inherit more clinically effective traditions of consultation than in the healthiest areas; and hospital doctors shoulder

heavier case-loads with less staff and equipment, more obsolete buildings, and suffer recurrent crises in the availability of beds and replacement staff. These trends can be summed up as the inverse care law: that the availability of good medical care tends to vary inversely with the need of the population served.

(Hart 1971)

At the time, evidence certainly existed to back this claim. One study found that in predominantly working-class areas, 80 per cent of GP surgeries were built before 1900 compared to less than 50 per cent in middle-class areas, where 25 per cent had been built since 1945 (Cartwright and Marshall 1965). This was despite the fact that the founders of the National Health Service were unambiguous about a desire to achieve greater equality. Speaking in the House of Commons in 1946, the Minister of Health, Aneurin Bevan, announced: 'we have got to achieve as nearly as possible a uniform standard of service for all – only with a national health service can the state ensure that an equally good service is available everywhere' (Quoted in Allsop, 1984).

However, the service emerged from an array of service provision that was far from equitable. Better-off areas often had more services available to them, and opportunities to access specialist services varied enormously across the country. For much of the early history of the NHS, patterns of provision reflected those established in the pre-NHS era. In 1971–2, hospital spending per head of the population in one region was 41 per cent higher than the average, while in another region it was 23 per cent below, a disparity that could not be explained by variations in clinical need. A 1972 study found that Newcastle, for example, had twice as many gynaecologists for every adult female in the city compared to Sheffield. The ratio of consultants to the population was twice as high in Birmingham as in Sheffield (Cooper and Culyer 1972).

Richard Crossman, the Health Minister at the time, described the problem of dealing with relatively disadvantaged regions as the most difficult he had to face (Allsop 1984: 93) and during the 1970s considerable effort was expended in tackling regional resource inequalities. New funding formulae were introduced, intended to match resources to indicators of current need, rather than being based on past patterns of spending.

While not entirely removed, many of the inequities in premises and equipment were addressed as a consequence. But evidence of variations in the use being made of services, between the better and worse off, continued to mount. Richard Titmuss, writing in 1968, claimed:

We have learnt from fifteen years' experience of the Health Service that the higher income groups know how to make better use of the service; they tend to receive more specialist attention; occupy more of the beds in better equipped and staffed hospitals; receive more elective surgery; have better maternal care and are more likely to get psychiatric help and psychotherapy than low-income groups – particularly the unskilled.

(Titmuss 1968, in Butterworth and Weir 1976: 476)

Progress may have been made in addressing the inequitable distribution of resources but this did not seem to have removed inequities in the use of the services being provided. If choice in health care is to have real meaning, this is a feature to be explored and explained.

Are health services accessed equitably?

Before examining examples of evidence drawn from studies focusing on specific conditions and treatments, it may be helpful to consider a much broader question. Who gets most from the NHS? There is evidence to suggest that poorer people now receive more services than do the better off: does this suggest that the problems of unequal access have been resolved? One way to approach this is to measure what is sometimes described as the 'social wage', taking account of benefits received from welfare services and not simply from income.

Tom Sefton, of the Economic and Social Research Council's Centre for Analysis of Social Exclusion, has looked at the amount of health care spending directed to the poorest fifth (or quintile) of the population, the second poorest fifth, and so on through to the wealthiest fifth. He takes account of the fact that age and gender differences within each of these groups will explain some of the differences: for example, men aged over 75 are twice as likely to have an outpatient appointment as men aged 35–55, and women have 50 per cent more GP consultations than do men. The table below shows the share of health care received by each income group (column 1) and that which they might expect to receive if based on their age and sex (column 2). Column 3 represents the difference between the actual and expected share in each case, with a positive number indicating a receipt of service greater than would be expected on demographic characteristics.

Table 10.1 Distribution of health care benefits 2000/01

	Actual share received (1)	Share received if based on age and gender (2)	Income effect (1)–(2)
Bottom quintile	23.2%	21.8%	+1.4%
Second quintile	27.2%	22.9%	+4.3%
Third quintile	21.0%	20.0%	+1.0%
Fourth quintile	16.0%	18.1%	−2.1%
Top quintile	12.6%	17.2%	−4.6%

Source: Sefton (2000)

The table shows the poorest fifth of the population receive 1.4 per cent more resources than age and gender composition would predict as an equitable allocation, while the second poorest fifth does even better, gaining 4.3 per cent more than would be suggested by these demographic factors. In contrast, the wealthiest fifth has 4.6 per cent less spent on it than might be anticipated. The study's author concludes:

> The overall distribution of health care benefits in kind is pro-poor, but with a clear hump in the distribution. Those in the second quintile group receive more than those in the bottom income group, but both groups receive substantially more than higher income groups. This pro-poor bias appears consistently across different health care services.
>
> (Sefton 2000: 24)

However, although this takes account of variations in anticipated clinical need associated with the demographic characteristics of age and sex, it does not incorporate an equivalent adjustment for social characteristics, such as those related to housing and employment. As was shown in previous chapters, these are factors closely associated with differences in health status.

It is important to know whether the greater use made of the health service by poorer people is equivalent to the higher incidence of illness they experience. If the two are approximately the same this might be strong grounds for believing that services are accessed equitably. If, on the other hand, the excess of illness among poorer groups exceeds their extra use of health care, a different conclusion must be drawn.

Several sources of data on levels of illness or morbidity exist, although each has limitations. For example, NHS statistics count only those actually in receipt of services, which will not throw much light on the question of how much untreated illness exists. Possible alternative data sources are the census and other surveys, particularly the General Household Survey (GHS) and the Health Survey for England. Each of these includes questions about illness, with the census having the advantage that it covers the whole of the population rather than a representative sample. However, a benefit of the other surveys is that respondents are also asked about their use of the health service during the preceding year.

Analysing GHS data on morbidity and GP attendance for the years 1971 to 1976 the Black Report concluded: 'The data are limited and further analyses remain to be carried out, but what is available suggests that the level of consultation among partly skilled and unskilled manual workers does not appear to match their need for health care' (Townsend and Davidson 1982: 79–80).

In addition to the ratio of the number of consultations to levels of need, the report also drew attention to studies on the quality of interactions:

> Several studies have shown that middle-class patients tend to have longer consultations than working-class patients and that more problems are discussed during this period. One study also found that middle-class patients were able to make better use of the consultation time, as measured by the number of items of information communicated, and the number of questions asked. Moreover, even though working-class patients tended to have been with the practice for longer, the doctors seemed to have more knowledge of the

personal and domestic circumstances of their middle-class patients. An earlier study found, for example, that middle-class patients were more likely to be visited by their GP when in hospital than were working-class patients. For cultural reasons, then, and also because there is a tendency for the 'better' doctors to work in middle-class areas, the suggestion must be that middle-class patients appear to receive a better service when they do present themselves than their working-class contemporaries.

(Townsend and Davidson 1982: 78–79)

Turning to hospital services, the Black Report noted that data was more limited but that which existed: 'suggest that the rate of usage of hospital beds rises with declining class. In Scotland, an analysis of hospital admission rates and duration of stay found clear upwards trends in both with declining class' (Townsend and Davidson 1982: 80–81).

The report also expressed concern that: 'Inequalities appear to be greatest (and most worrying) in the case of the preventative services. Severe under-utilization by the working classes is a complex result of under-provision, of costs (financial, psychological) of attendance, and perhaps of a life-style which profoundly inhibits any attempt at rational action in the interests of *future* well-being' (Townsend and Davidson 1982: 88).

The conclusion reached in the report on the whole issue of inequalities in the use of the health service is worth quoting in full:

It is hard to resist the conclusion that this pattern of unequal use is explicable not in terms of non-rational response to sickness by working-class people, but of a rational weighting of the perceived costs and benefits to them of attendance and compliance with the prescribed regime. These costs and benefits differ between the social classes both on account of differences in way of life, constraints and resources, and of the fact that costs to the working class are actually increased by the lower levels and perhaps poorer quality of provision to which many have access.

Class differentials in the use of various services which we have considered derive from the interaction of social and ecological factors. Differences in sheer availability and, at least to some extent, in the quality of care available in different *localities* provide one channel by which social inequality permeates the NHS. Reduced provision implied greater journeys, longer waiting lists, longer waiting times, difficulties in obtaining an appointment, shortage of space and so on. A second channel is provided by the structuring of health care *institutions* in accordance with the values, assumptions and preferences of the sophisticated middle-class 'consumer'. Inadequate attention may be paid to the different problems and needs of those who are less able to express themselves in acceptable terms and who suffer from lack of command over resources both of time and of money. In all cases, for an individual to seek medical care, his (or her) perception of his (or her) need for care will have to outweigh the perceived costs (financial and other) both of seeking care and of the regime which may be prescribed. These costs are class related.

(Townsend and Davidson 1982: 89)

Observing that inequalities in health care access arise from the interaction between these two sets of factors, the report poses a question of continuing relevance. How far, then, has the situation changed since the 1970s? In *The Health Divide*, Margaret Whitehead reviewed later evidence, which included several examples of studies suggesting that better-off patients were more likely to receive specialist care. She also notes that the relationship between GP use and clinical need is a highly complex one but that evidence showed manual groups made more use of GP services than did non-manual groups. This led one study published in 1980, but using data from 1974, to conclude: 'the NHS has achieved equity in terms of access to primary health care'.

Although this study was criticized on several grounds, a subsequent reanalysis of the same data by the OPCS confirmed that:

For given rates of sickness those in the manual socio-economic groups were more likely to consult a GP than those in the non-manual groups. The result was clearer for acute than for chronic sickness and more marked for men than for women. The conclusion was that, from 1974 data, 'for the aspect studied there was no evidence of bias'.

(Whitehead 1992: 282)

With other colleagues, Whitehead has continued to examine this issue and in 1997 published further analysis using GHS data, comparing periods from the mid-1980s to the mid-1990s. Starting with self-reported health status, in the mid-1908s the data shows statistically significant differences between occupational groups:

Table 10.2 Percentage of respondents reporting fair or poor health (Great Britain)

	1984–5	1990–1	1993–4
Professional	21.8	19.3	27.2
Unskilled manual	45.2	47.0	47.2

Source: Whitehead et al. (1997)

We can compare these changes with data on GP consultations and outpatient appointments during the same time period. In the mid-1980s there was little difference in rates of GP consultation by professional and unskilled manual workers but by the 1990s unskilled manual workers were considerably more likely to consult with their GP. This is shown in the following figures, using odds ratios, a way of comparing whether the probability of an event is the same for different groups. Numbers higher than one indicate a greater probability and vice versa.

Table 10.3 Consultations with general practitioners

	1984–5	1990–1	1993–4
Professional	1.00	1.00	1.00
Unskilled manual	1.07	1.36	1.41

Source: Whitehead *et al.* (1997)

Ratios shown have been adjusted to take account of variations between groups in age and other relevant factors.

In other words, if it was the case in the past that working-class patients were less likely to visit their GP, relative to the amount of sickness experienced, such a gap seems to have reduced substantially during these years. This was also a period during which many manual occupations experienced substantial cuts in jobs, as traditional industries went into decline. Mention has previously been made of political controversies over the use of sickness and incapacity benefit to conceal unemployment figures, raising an intriguing possibility that increased contact with the health system may have been encouraged by the state. Whatever the case for this, and data is simply too limited to adequately explain the increasing consultation of manual workers with GPs, this trend was not reflected in outpatient visits. Although there was a small increase in appointments among manual workers, there was no statistically significant difference between the two occupational groups during this same period.

Table 10.4 Outpatient visits

	1984–85	1990–1	1993–4
Professional	1.00	1.00	1.00
Unskilled manual	0.85	1.02	0.93

Source: Whitehead *et al.* (1997)

In summary, the three tables above suggest that in 1993–4 the proportion of unskilled manual workers who reported having 'fair' or 'poor' health was 74 per cent higher than among professional workers but this translated into only 40 per cent more GP consultations. In addition, unskilled manual workers were no more likely than professional workers to receive an outpatient department appointment.

This conclusion is broadly supported by an analysis of data from the Health Survey for England, covering the period 1994 to 1999. A review of this study summarizes the findings as follows:

> lower income individuals were less likely to have inpatient treatment than higher income ones; the unemployed were less likely to have outpatient

treatment; and those with lower educational attainment were less likely to have outpatient, day case and inpatient treatment.

(Dixon *et al.* 2003: 11)

The researchers conclude that health care needs do not seem to translate directly into use of health services:

After controlling for morbidity in a number of dimensions, more deprived individuals (in terms of income, education and employment) have lower than expected use of health services. This implies that there may be unmet need for health care in terms of income, employment and educational deprivation.

(Sutton *et al.* cited in Dixon *et al.* 2003: 11)

Inequalities in chronic illness

A distinction that has emerged previously is the one between acute and chronic illness. Data from the General Household Survey (GHS) allows some comparison of episodes of acute sickness and experiences of chronic illness between socio-economic groups, although direct comparison with earlier statistics is limited by the changes in categories that are used (these were described in Chapter 7). In the table below these categories are used to show data from the 2001 General Household Survey. Columns (1) to (3) show the proportion of each employment category reporting chronic sickness, acute sickness and having consulted a GP in the preceding two weeks. In light of the 1974 data, showing that increased rates of GP consultation among manual groups were more marked for acute sickness than for chronic sickness, separate ratios are shown of GP consultations to rates of acute and chronic sickness in columns (4) and (5).

This data suggests that workers in routine occupations were around 50 per cent more likely than were large employers and those in higher managerial occupations to have experienced acute sickness in the 14 days before the interview. There is a very similar differential in the likelihood of having consulted a GP in that same period.

There are also some striking differences between chronic and acute sickness. Two aspects are particularly apparent. First, socio-economic inequalities in experiences of health are wider for chronic sickness than for acute sickness: when asked about limiting long-term illness, routine workers were more than twice as likely to suffer in comparison to those in higher managerial positions. Second, these wider inequalities are not reflected clearly in extra GP consultations, in contrast to the ratio of acute sickness to GP consultation, which shows little difference by socio-economic group. It may also be worth noting that 71 per cent of male routine and manual workers received a prescription, compared to 57 per cent of managerial and professional patients.

Earlier chapters have described some of the evidence that suggests a role for psychosocial factors in the aetiology of chronic illness. Data of the kind available from sources such as the GHS appear to confirm the occupational class gradient found by researchers such as Michael Marmot in relation to coronary heart

Table 10.5 Self-reported sickness and GP consultations (males)

	(1) Chronic sickness	(2) Acute sickness	(3) GP consultation	(4) Ratio of GP consultations to chronic sickness	(5) Ratio of GP consultations to acute sickness
Large employers and higher managerial	13%	12%	10%	0.77	0.83
Higher professional	12%	11%	10%	0.83	0.91
Lower managerial and professional	15%	11%	9%	0.6	0.82
Intermediate	16%	9%	10%	0.63	1.11
Small employers and own account	17%	12%	11%	0.65	0.92
Lower supervisory and technical	21%	15%	13%	0.62	0.87
Semi-routine	21%	13%	12%	0.57	0.92
Routine	27%	17%	15%	0.55	0.88
Long-term unemployed	22%	17%	14%	0.64	0.82

Source: Sheaff (2003)

disease. However, unequal experiences of chronic illness do not appear to be matched by an equivalent increase in the use of primary health care.

The term chronic illness covers a wide range of conditions, which are long-term and bring some degree of incapacity or suffering. On this definition, it incorporates conditions as diverse as coronary heart disease, diabetes, chronic respiratory problems and arthritis. The list is very similar to the types of illnesses that attracted the attention of Halliday in the 1930s and 1940s (see Chapter 6). As the list is so extensive, it is impossible to comment adequately on all aspects in this review but in an effort to do justice to questions prompted by the data, the following section provides a selective focus on coronary heart disease to discuss inequalities in the use of health services.

The case of coronary heart disease

In her review of research evidence on health inequalities in the late 1980s, Whitehead refers to research by Findlay that appeared to show poorer patients received less medical intervention for heart disease:

A study in Glasgow found that clinical investigations for heart disease (coronary angiography) were performed more frequently on patients from more affluent neighbourhoods. The men with the lowest level of deprivation had only half the expected death rates from heart disease, but one and a half times their predicted rates of angiographies. In contrast, men in the most deprived areas had death rates one-third higher than average, with only three-quarters of the predicted rate of investigation. A similar pattern emerged for women and raised the question of whether doctors fail to refer or investigate these patients sufficiently.

(Whitehead 1992: 279–80)

More recently, two valuable reviews of evidence on inequalities in access to health care have given some attention to studies dealing with coronary heart disease and cardiac care services (Goddard and Smith 2001; Dixon *et al.* 2003). Goddard and Smith conclude that:

the weight of evidence relating to the treatment of coronary heart disease suggests that admissions, rates of investigation and revascularisation do not match the higher levels of need experienced by the most disadvantaged groups compared with more affluent groups.

(Goddard and Smith 2001: 1157)

However, not all work in this area points to an incontrovertible or unanimous conclusion. The following provides a summary of some of the studies, including possible explanations that have been put forward to account for the findings. Different results may simply reflect variable local circumstances, something which cannot easily be determined by comparing separate local studies. Nevertheless, the data prompts several interesting and important questions.

Some useful data comes from a large-scale Scottish study, based on 307,741 patients registered with general practices participating in the Scottish continuing morbidity recording project. Of this total number of patients, 2186 were seen at least once for heart failure between April 1999 and March 2000. These patients received a total of 5285 GP consultations during the year, representing a mean number of contacts of 2.4.

Examining the data, the authors note:

The incidence of heart failure significantly increased with increasing social deprivation: socioeconomically deprived patients were 44 per cent more likely to develop heart failure than affluent patients. In contrast, the association between socioeconomic deprivation and contacts or consultation was in the opposite direction: patients in the most deprived groups had 23 per cent fewer follow up visits each year with their general practitioner.

Socioeconomically deprived individuals are more likely to develop heart failure but less likely to see their general practitioner on an ongoing basis.

(McAlister *et al.* 2004)

The authors consider a number of possible explanations for this finding. First, it might be that individuals from more economically deprived groups are more fatalistic, with greater expectation of being ill, and more likely to seek advice from non-professionals. Second, there is data to suggest that those from deprived areas are more likely to seek and receive care in accident and emergency departments than in primary care. Evidence to support this has been found in studies of other cardiovascular and respiratory illnesses 'characterised by intermittent acute exacerbations' (Blatchford *et al.* 1999), which may also relate to evidence described in Chapter 4 on how individuals interpret and act upon symptoms. This might provide an important pointer to interpreting the sometimes conflicting evidence on inequalities in the use of health services. Choices made about when and how to access services are rarely isolated, individual decisions but more frequently represent the end point of a series of personal and social influences.

A third potential explanation considered in this study was that GPs may be less likely to offer follow-up care for some groups of patients; in this case, those from more economically deprived backgrounds. However, there was no evidence of any statistically significant variation in issuing prescriptions between more and less affluent groups (McAlister *et al.* 2004).

These need not be alternative explanations and it may be that they operate and interact to produce the reduced number of follow-up visits among poorer patients. Whatever the precise causes, other studies suggest that better-off patients are more likely to make use of cardiac services.

A study conducted in Sheffield examined the relationship between deprivation and revascularization using data from a sample of 491 people with angina symptoms. The authors found that: 'deprived wards had only about half the numbers of revascularisations per head of population estimated to have angina symptoms than did affluent wards' (Payne and Saul 1997).

Similarly, an examination of angiography rates showed that 11.2 per cent of the sample in the ten most affluent wards had received an angiography, compared to 4.2 per cent in the ten most deprived wards.

The authors conclude:

Our results show a large local variation in both mortality from coronary heart disease and prevalence of angina as determined by a population survey. Both mortality and prevalence of symptoms were strongly correlated with material deprivation, as estimated by the Townsend score, at electoral ward level. We found that the ratio of rates of coronary artery revascularisation to the prevalence of angina symptom varied substantially across the city and was inversely proportional to deprivation. Thus, use of services was not commensurate with need and seemed to exhibit the inverse care law, even though the availability of care is the same.

(Payne and Saul 1997)

However, a slightly more complex picture emerges from a study of variations in the use of specialist cardiac services in the North-West of England. This examined the utilization of the diagnostic technique of coronary angiography (also known as catheterization) and revascularization using CABG or PTCA: 'The general conclusion is that, for angiography and CABG interventions there is evidence of an increase in the rate of investigation as deprivation increases but not for PTCAs' (Gatrell *et al.* 2002: 150).

It may be that in addition to the possibility of local variations, other factors, including age and gender, play a part in producing this outcome. A study of CABG revascularization rates in the area covered by what was then the North East Thames Regional Health Authority offers some support to this hypothesis (Ben-Shlomo and Chaturvedi 1995). Unsurprisingly, a steady increase in rates of ischaemic heart disease was associated with increasing area scores for deprivation. This applied to both men and women. For women, CABG rates tended to follow the mortality trends, indicating a more or less equitable provision of health care. Assuming mortality rates provide a reliable guide to overall prevalence, a reasonably close correspondence between these and therapeutic interventions imply the latter are being appropriately targeted.

Yet this relationship did not hold for men. Here the researchers found what they describe as a 'U' relationship between rates of CABG and measures of deprivation. Lower rates of CABG were found among men in the second and third quartiles of deprivation, that is, those in the 'middle' categories. Had rates matched those for mortality, as was the case for women, it would be expected that these would have been higher than those for men in the first quartile (the most affluent). This was not the case. However, the highest rates of CABG operations were carried out on men living in the most deprived areas, accurately reflecting rates of disease. These men also tended to live closest to the hospitals where the procedures were carried out.

Several of the studies described here were carried out in the 1990s, and many changes in health care have occurred since that time. Dixon et al. (2003) suggest that the introduction of the Coronary Heart Disease National Service Framework may be stimulating the development of more equitable arrangements:

> The investment in CHD services and emphasis on identifying and treating need based on clear clinical guidelines has certainly altered the quantum of CHD care available and may have altered its distribution. Further research would be valuable to confirm this.
>
> (Dixon et al. 2003: 13)

It is probably too early to reach a judgement on this but there is one further feature of the studies described here that merits attention: the use made of primary care services by different socio-economic groups. One possible explanation for the lack of total consistency between findings might be that patterns of primary and secondary care intervention differ. It might be, for example, that more deprived groups use more acute hospital services. However, this is a consequence of more limited intervention at an earlier stage, which might have made some of this unnecessary. The possibility that this may be a factor is raised in one research project, examining health service utilization at the level of general practices. (Asthana et al. no date).

The aim of the study was to examine variations in health service utilization according to need, using data from 12 contrasting health authority areas. Census-derived information on self-reported illness and socio-economic status was combined with other data to generate measures of health care needs, which were then compared with indicators of health service use, including data on prescriptions, referrals and admissions for specific conditions.

The data were based on the activity of over 550 general practices serving a population of 3.5 million patients, and the researchers note:

> Some of our findings are at odds with the received wisdom that the use of NHS services is characterised by an inverse care law. For example, examining use in relation to need for cardiology services, urban practices that are close to acute hospitals and whose practice populations are highly biased in service uptake holds when factors such as demography, service accessibility and rurality are controlled for.
>
> (Asthana *et al.* no date)

However, the authors go on to comment:

> The assumption that higher rates of hospital care are necessarily a 'good thing' should also be revisited. Within the urban setting, the pro-poor bias in levels of hospitalisation may reflect poorer primary and community management, suggesting a need for a stronger public health focus.

This line of argument receives support from a range of studies that show patients from deprived socio-economic groups are more likely than those from affluent groups to experience emergency admission to hospital care. It is also worth noting that most studies of hospital treatment include inpatients, rather than day patients who now comprise two-thirds of all surgical patients. This means that emergency admissions are likely to be disproportionately represented among inpatients (Dixon *et al.* 2003: 19).

This suggests the importance of the complete 'care pathway' when comparing rates of access between socio-economic groups. Having higher rates of emergency admissions among poorer groups might justify describing the NHS as 'pro-poor', however, this may be a consequence of more limited primary care utilization. Rushing people into hospital with blue lights flashing is an unfortunate means of achieving equity.

Inequality and seeking professional help

Responding to research findings of this type requires that attention is given to how individuals make decisions about contacting the health service. To gain a better understanding of the factors that may be involved in creating differences it is important to explore people's own experiences and accounts, for which qualitative studies can be more appropriate than quantitative data. These enable people to express their own views and feelings, not restricted to the format of a pre-deter-mined questionnaire. A consequence is that research of this kind often involves quite small numbers, which can make generalization from the findings difficult. Nevertheless, qualitative studies provide important insights into people's own experiences.

Work in this area includes Tod *et al.* (2001) who examined the experiences of 14 patients and nine primary care staff through interviews. Obstacles to making full use of services identified in the interviews were placed into six categories:

1. Structural factors – e.g. poor transport, inconvenient surgery times
2. Personal factors – e.g. fear and denial of illness
3. Social and cultural factors – e.g. value placed on coping and strength
4. Past experiences and expectations – e.g. poor experience of health service
5. Diagnostic confusion – e.g. chest pains not attributed to heart
6. Knowledge and awareness – e.g. poor understanding of heart disease

Examples of statements made by respondents' interviews provide a guide to the issues involved. From patients:

> You think it'll go off. I think a lot of people, they think, well what I don't know won't hurt me.

> People from round here cope. They don't like making a fuss. They have a depth of character.

> And I get these pains and they tell me, like, with having this arthritis and that and dust, you see, you can get pains through your chest with arthritis and I can get pains in my chest with the dust – so I don't know whether I'm coming or going.

And from primary care staff:

> Patients will be getting angina on a daily basis and … they brush it off. It's almost par for the course. I'm astonished at their laid backness about this.

> It is easy to attribute pain to the chest rather than recognise it as angina, so I think patients in this area are at a disadvantage, because they probably blame their symptoms rather on their lungs and their chest than their heart … I'm sure people delay a lot because they think it is their chest and if it doesn't resolve they might come to the doctor.

> (Tod *et al.* 2001)

See also Gardner, Chapple and Green (1999) who also looked at barriers to referral in patients with angina, interviewing 16 patients and their doctors in Toxteth, Liverpool.

A study in Glasgow, based on interviews with 30 people from an affluent area and 30 from a deprived area, found people were more likely to perceive themselves as being at risk of heart disease when they had experiences of it among family members, and these people felt a stronger identification with groups at high risk of heart disease (Richards, Reid and Watt 2002). This tended to be more common among those from more deprived areas. However, this greater perceived vulnerability was not associated with more frequent consultations with a GP:

People from the deprived area reported greater exposure to ill health, which allowed them to normalise their chest pain, led to confusion with other conditions, and gave rise to a belief that they were overusing medical services ... Anxiety about presenting among respondents in the deprived area was heightened by self-blame and fear that they would be chastened by their general practitioner for their risk behaviours.

(Richards, Reid and Watt 2002: 1308)

These studies suggest that evidence of an inverse relationship between need and use of health services is not always associated with inequitable provision of facilities. Access to services requires more than their physical availability and the way in which they are provided, and how these two elements are perceived, can be as important as geography in constructing obstacles to access.

There is also recent data that suggests different social groups do not receive the same level of attention during consultations. Stirling's study of GP consultations in the West of Scotland found average lengths of 8.7 minutes. However, while the two most affluent groups received between 9.5 and 10.25 minutes, the average for the others was around 8 to 8.5 minutes (Stirling, Wilson and McConnachie 2001).

Attention so far has focused on what might be regarded as social class inequalities in access to health services but another important source is ethnic origin. Issues arising from cultural expectations and assumptions can create significant differences in outcomes. One consequence can be what Goffman described as the 'tribal stigma' of race and nationality, generating the potential for unequal and discriminatory responses. This may not entail overt or explicit racism, but can be evident in what has come to be described as 'institutional racism'.

Ethnicity, health care and 'institutional racism'

The term institutional racism gained prominence as a result of the inquiry by the Metropolitan Police into the investigation of the murder of black teenager, Stephen Lawrence. The inquiry, reporting in 1999, provides the following definition:

Institutional racism is the collective failure of an organisation to provide an appropriate and professional service to people because of their colour, culture or ethnic origin. It can be seen or detected in processes, attitudes and behaviour which amount to discrimination through unwitting prejudice, ignorance, thoughtlessness and racist stereotyping, which disadvantage minority ethnic people.

(MacPherson 1999)

This definition, sometimes referred to as the MacPherson definition, after William MacPherson who chaired the Stephen Lawrence inquiry, does not require overtly racist behaviour. Use of the words 'unwitting' and 'ignorance' emphasize that its focus is upon a lack of attention to cultural differences, having the effect of being discriminatory whether or not this is the intention. Although the context of the Lawrence inquiry was the policing of a criminal investigation, its approach was incorporated into another more recent inquiry into aspects of NHS provision.

This inquiry was established following the death of David "Rocky" Bennett, an African-Caribbean who suffered from schizophrenia and had been receiving NHS treatment for 18 years. On the evening of his death, David Bennett had been racially abused by another patient, who was white. Each of the men struck each other, and following this incident, David Bennett was moved to another ward in the unit.

On the new ward, he hit a nurse, leading to him being restrained by a group of nurses which resulted in a struggle. During this struggle, while being held face down on the floor, David Bennett collapsed and died.

Describing evidence that was presented to the inquiry, the subsequent report comments on remarks by one witness:

> Mr Francis had comments to make about racism which we found useful. He said that using the word 'racism' was not very helpful. It was necessary to deconstruct what racism was about. It was about human relationships and was based on power, namely the power of one person over another. Just using the word 'racism' did not communicate to people what it was that was discriminatory about what they did. To make things better it was necessary to explain that something was wrong with the relationship and to try and put it right.
>
> He therefore had some hesitation about the use of the term 'institutional racism', which he considered had its own complexities and its own history. But he told us that the sum total of his view was that the mental health services and the NHS were racist within the meaning of the McPherson definition of institutional racism. He emphasised that black patients were particularly sensitive to any hint of regulation, control or disrespect because they have been primed by their experiences to expect to be treated badly in society. (p. 43)

The inquiry report summarized much of the evidence that was heard:

> Many witnesses told us that the black and minority ethnic community have a very real fear of the Mental Health Service. They fear that if they engage with the mental health services they will be locked up for a long time, if not for life, and treated with medication which may eventually kill them ... Young black men with signs of mental illness frequently, out of fear, do not go to their doctor until their illness is so pronounced that their family and friends can no longer cope with them. By this time they tend to be isolated, not only from their own family but also from their own peer group. Their illness is by then more difficult to treat and treatment in the community may not be a real option.
>
> (Blofield 2003)

This again points to the importance of understanding how decisions and choices made by individuals are shaped by prior experiences and expectations. Pilgrim and Rogers (1993) discuss the over-representation of African-Caribbeans with schizophrenia, and the under-representation of Asian groups, in terms of three types of explanation. The first focuses on 'cultural difference'. However, this can be interpreted in different ways: for example, either that lower rates of distress among Asian communities reflects psychological robustness, or higher levels of stigma. A second type of explanation emphasizes the effect of the environment, although Pilgrim and Rogers point out that many Asians experience disadvantage and racism.

A third explanation connects with the issues raised in the inquiry into the death of Rocky Bennett: the response of psychiatric services, and others involved with them, to black people. For example, higher proportions of black people are referred to these services by police and magistrates (Pilgrim and Rogers 1993).

Stereotyping behaviour

A different context provides another example of the ways assumptions about behaviour can influence outcomes. It is not only the perceptions of patients that influence how services are used. Health care staff may also make assumptions about the likely behaviour of patients which, in some circumstances, can become something of a self-fulfilling prophecy.

The example to be used arises from a study examining genetic screening for thalassaemia, a genetic blood disorder (Modell *et al.* 2000). Each year at least 75,000 infants are born to women in ethnic groups at risk of haemoglobin disorders, with about 7000 of these women carrying the disorder, in addition to nearly 1000 of their partners. Screening can be offered to expectant mothers to detect if the embryo has the disorder.

Prenatal screening, which may result in the termination of a pregnancy, raises controversial issues, but as a service offered within the NHS would presumably be available equitably to all mothers who might be at risk. A national audit of 138 women who had a pregnancy affected by thalassaemia between 1990 and 1994 indicates this may not be so. Together, the 138 women had a total of 485 pregnancies, 85 of which were ineligible (because of miscarriage, occurring before prenatal screening was available, or some other reason). For the remaining 400 pregnancies, the table below shows the percentage of occasions on which the couple were offered prenatal diagnosis, by ethnic group.

How are such wide variations in the proportions of each ethnic group offered the diagnosis to be explained? Factors include geographical variations in the availability of facilities, however, it also appears that there are variations in the extent to which these facilities were sought by different ethnic groups:

British Cypriots are highly aware of thalassaemia and have high expectations; many 'beat the system' by asking their doctor for prepregnancy screening and so obtain prenatal diagnosis in the first trimester of their first pregnancy. By contrast, most British Pakistanis depend on health workers for information and

Table 10.6 Percentage of couples offered prenatal diagnosis, by ethnic group

Ethnic group	% offered prenatal diagnosis
Cypriot	92%
Indian	63%
Other	61%
Pakistani	51%
Bangladeshi	35%
Total	67%

Source: Modell *et al.* (2000)

screening and few know that prenatal diagnosis in the first trimester is available with religious agreement in Pakistan and Iran. We show here that British Pakistanis' low utilisation of prenatal diagnosis reflects inadequate risk detection, lack of awareness, poor communication, and a strong preference for early testing. It is, however, often taken to support a view (documented in several notes) that Muslims 'do not want' prenatal diagnosis. This leads to half-hearted screening and self-confirming results, so the population that needs the best service obtains the worst.

The eight British Bangladeshi couples studied encountered most problems. There was no evidence of any counselling for four couples, no couple was counselled in their mother tongue, and two couples at risk of haemoglobin E/- thalassaemia were not offered prenatal diagnosis because their risk was incorrectly assessed. Although two haemoglobinopathy counsellors with appropriate language skills are in post in the United Kingdom, they are geo-graphically inaccessible to most British Bangladeshis.

(Model *et al.* 2000: 340)

The stage of pregnancy when screening was offered also contributed to variations in outcomes. The authors note:

The choices of British Pakistanis highlight the importance of the timing of offering prenatal diagnosis. In this group, uptake of prenatal diagnosis in the first trimester is over 70 per cent and over 90 per cent of affected pregnancies are terminated, whereas uptake of diagnosis in the second trimester is 40 per cent and half of the affected pregnancies are terminated. The same preference applies for couples of any ethnic origin but is often masked by higher acceptance of late abortion. Informed choice clearly requires the offer of diagnosis in the first trimester whenever possible, which will require increased involvement of primary care teams.

(p. 340)

Cultural traditions can have a profound effect on individual decisions and a failure to acknowledge their importance risks contributing to unjustifiable differences in services accessed by different ethnic groups. Again, it demonstrates how equality of access requires more than the physical availability of services.

Health care: making a difference

Although examples of inadequate provision in deprived areas remain, most evidence points to substantial improvements in the physical distribution of facilities since the 1960s and 1970s. Problems arising from a lack of transport, however, continue to be experienced by many patients. A study conducted in a paediatric clinic in Leeds found that 63 per cent of children attending had come by car, whereas only 37 per cent of those failing to attend had access to a car, with the majority having to rely on public transport or walking (McClure, Newell and Edwards 1996).

A discussion on the question of whether extending greater choice to patients will worsen or reduce health inequalities gives attention to the role access to transport plays:

> An essential element of any policy aimed at encouraging choice is the provision of help with transport and travel costs. This might involve better planning of public transport infrastructures and timetables to enable easier access to a range of health facilities at all times or by patient transportation arrangements made on behalf of the patients by the NHS. Ideally, financial help would cover the full range of costs, including the costs of time off work and costs associated with an accompanying partner or carer. If the policy were an extension of the existing hospital travel costs scheme it would be targeted on patients who are in receipt of income support, income based jobseeker's allowance, pension credit, working tax credit and/or child tax credit and those assessed as low income or who have to travel frequently over long distances.
>
> (Le Grand and Dixon 2004: 9–10)

Adequate transport represents an essential and fundamental element of improving access to health services, but without disregarding or underestimating its importance, it need not be addressed in detail here. A key focus of this book has been upon the social relationship between patients and professionals, and the institutional setting within which care is delivered. It is these aspects, therefore, that provide a conclusion to this chapter.

Inequalities between professionals and patients in general were considered in earlier chapters, with attention given to what this can mean for communication between the two. Mention was made in Chapter 5 of research by Kennedy *et al.* that suggested the provision of information to patients did not necessarily alter choice but could do so when accompanied by a structured interview with a nurse. It did not seem that this simply was a result of improved information but, to repeat the conclusion from the study, the involvement of a nurse helped women to get what they wanted. Other women knew what they wanted, 'but they seemed less able to communicate their preference to the gynaecologist' (Kennedy *et al.* 2002: 21).

This reflects a generalized imbalance of authority between the professional and the patient. In this example, the role of the nurse was important as a counterbalance to the inequality between patient and doctor. But, as we have seen, the level of inequality between patient and professional is not only a consequence of that particular relationship but is also the product of wider social divisions.

Dixon *et al.* (2003) adopt the term 'voice', from a contrast used by Hirschman (1970) between this and 'exit' as a means of dealing with difficulties, to explore the idea that middle-class patients are more effective at expressing their needs and having them met. This may reflect the smaller social distance between them and professionals such as doctors, and the fact that social connections between them, their families and friends are more likely than for those engaged in manual work. Such connections need not be direct and immediate for them to have an effect. As has been noted, there is research to indicate that the length and quality of the consultation can vary between social classes, and although Dixon *et al.* note this is limited, other corroborative evidence suggests a similar conclusion:

> More direct evidence of the exact mechanisms through which voice operates would be desirable. However, when such evidence as does exist is taken together with the indirect but well established evidence showing marked differences in referral rates and other treatments relative to need, it is likely that differences in the ability of social groups to express their voice is a major factor affecting differential success.
>
> (Dixon *et al.* 2003: 26)

If it is correct to conclude that societal inequalities reinforce the effects of the unequal relationship between patients and professionals, some practical implications can be identified fairly readily. Some are suggested by Dixon *et al.* in comments on what is identified as the most significant action required for reducing remaining inequalities in the use of health care:

> The challenge now for government is to find ways of addressing the remaining barriers to access: those connected with differences between social groups in respect of strength of 'voice' and in their health beliefs and health seeking behaviour. Several aspects of the current choice agenda have the potential to address these. Already in the London Choice Pilot, patients have been supported to exercise choice to move to another provider for quicker treatment . . . Choice is being offered as a matter of course to all (clinically eligible) patients and is supported with information and a patient care adviser.
>
> (Dixon *et al.* 2003: 30)

Enabling choice for patients

Significantly, the authors also note that preliminary analysis of the data suggests there is no relationship between deprivation and choice. In other words, patients from more deprived neighbourhoods were as likely to exercise choice as those living in more affluent areas. If confirmed, this would challenge assumptions that extensions to choice are inevitably likely to favour the middle class, thereby disadvantaging the least well off. Dixon *et al.* believe that choice, when carefully introduced, has the potential to create the very opposite effect:

> Empowering all patients to make informed choices about their care (together with clinicians) could equalise the advantage that middle class patients currently exercise through their use of voice and connections. Higher quality and more tailored information delivered to patients at the time they need it could address the 'inverse information law'. Together with the right to exit (choice to move to another provider), this should improve the responsiveness of services and tackle negative perceptions of the NHS.
>
> (Dixon *et al.* 2003: 30)

Is this optimistic assessment justified? Before considering this question, it is helpful to follow through the argument as it is developed by Le Grand and Dixon (2004) in a proposal to create a new model of what they describe as 'guided' or 'supported' choice. The rationale for this lies in the evidence showing differing capacities between social groups to exercise effective choice, with the objective to 'level the playing field'. The thinking behind the model is described as arising from lessons of the London Choice Pilot, referred to above, in which patients were given choice about where their treatment would be delivered, and thus the time within which it could be carried out. The proposed model of guided or supported choice:

> would build on the highly successful Patient Care Adviser (PCA) experience in the choice pilots and the experience with other similar patient advocacy and support roles in the NHS. Responsibilities of this role could include monitoring care plans, offering choices of provider, discussing treatment options, identifying special needs regarding travel, disability (mobility) and language (communication), providing information and updates about the care pathway (including assessment, treatment and aftercare), booking appointments with providers, arranging transport, helping patients navigate the system, and supporting/coaching patients on self-care, self-management and behavioural change.
>
> (Le Grand and Dixon 2004: 12)

In part, what is being described is someone who can deal with the 'practicalities' of receiving treatment, and the writers are not prescriptive about how the role might be filled. Nurses, pharmacists and former patients (particularly in fields such as mental health) are mentioned, but this question introduces a possible difficulty:

> Depending on what model of support was implemented, one potential criticism is that it could be resource intensive. This would be especially likely if a

new professional role was created, generating an 'army of bureaucrats'. On the other hand, this would be less likely if it drew upon existing skills . . .

Care would have to be taken that the PCA did not become another layer of professional between the patient and the service, and also that the scheme did not encourage increased patient dependence. In this connection, it is worth noting that there are currently other positions in the NHS that fulfil some of the proposed PCA functions already, such as cancer nurse specialists, patient advocates, diabetic nurse specialists, NHS District Nurses, PALS staff, etc.

(Le Grand and Dixon 2004: 12–13)

Described in this way, the proposal is both simple and appealing. It would address some of the problems that have been identified as obstacles to achieving greater equity. There are, though, some important factors to consider about how this might be achieved.

One initial point, so obvious that it does not require elaboration here, is that a study into choice of treatment centre conducted in London will give patients a range of alternatives that may not be mirrored elsewhere in the country. Choice of where to have treatment may be far more constrained in large, rural regions.

Three other issues can be mentioned: treatment, time and place. The first concerns the form of choice that is made available. The London pilot provided patients with choice of alternative locations, including private providers as well as the NHS, but the treatment received would be broadly similar. In contrast, the study by Kennedy et al. (2002), described in Chapter 5, explored women's responses to being offered choice of intervention. These included less invasive options and it was apparent that choices varied under different conditions of support.

Extending choice to the treatment itself, and not only where it is received, is particularly relevant for chronic disease. To develop this, health care services would need to be considerably more flexible than at present. Without this the concept of choice would be in practice extremely limited. This issue also raises questions about the status and role of the person providing the advice and support. Some patient advocates might take a different view to the dominant medical one, creating the possibility of conflict; however, it is impossible to conceive of a genuine notion of choice that does not allow for this.

Making time for patients

If patients were to receive greater levels of guidance and support in making genuinely informed choices about which clinical intervention to accept, this would be likely to have repercussions for the operational delivery of services. This brings us to the second issue: time. If the provision of more active support for patients is to be incorporated into existing professional roles there are likely to be consequences for resources. But this is not the only factor to consider.

A study by James (1992), referred to in Chapter 9, includes an example of a nurse who, having worked previously in an acute hospital setting, moved to another job in a hospice. Soon after starting work in the hospice, the nurse describes feelings, when sitting by the bedside talking to patients, that she was not really working and that she ought to get on with some tasks. There is no point in ignoring the fact that many health care settings involve busy routines, which can get in the way of and undermine effective communication. Hospices were established in response to an identified need for environments better suited for terminally ill patients, for whom palliative care rather than curative treatment was appropriate.

It is unrealistic to imagine busy acute hospital wards could transform themselves easily into settings where communication is not limited or constrained. This presents challenges to the institutions involved, to address the management of competing demands. Waiting list targets and other similar performance indicators have tended to direct managerial attention towards the efficiency and productivity of the service, with the aim of achieving more treatments being dominant. There are good reasons for this but effective communication with patients can be a casualty.

Creating the right setting for patients

The third issue to mention is place. Not in the sense of choice of place of treatment, but the environment in which advice and support is provided. The effectiveness of this would be limited were it a hospital setting, by which time many choices determining this outcome will already have been made. Primary care would provide a more appropriate setting, in which an adviser is more likely to be brought into direct contact with a patient's personal and social circumstances. This might, in turn, require finding ways of addressing non-clinical needs, as was illustrated in the examples of locating welfare benefits advice in primary care, given in Chapter 6. Again, this raises questions about whether a health professional is most appropriate for this role.

Even the location of advice within a primary care setting is limited by the fact that patients contact a GP at different stages of an illness. Although, as we have seen, there is evidence to suggest inequalities in primary care access are declining more than is the case for outpatients, variations still remain. One option would be to move activity out of the formal health care setting into environments where those who are least likely to visit a doctor may be found.

It is known that those at most risk of illness are frequently those least likely to have contact with preventative and screening services. For example, a national study in the early 1990s, based on a 1 per cent sample of all GP lists in England and Wales, found that adults aged 16–44 in unskilled and semi-skilled manual occupations were 10 per cent less likely to have had consultations for preventative health care than those in professional and intermediate occupations (McCormick, Fleming and Charlton 1995).

Several initiatives have been introduced in an attempt to address this problem. One example of a project designed to bring health care out of a narrow clinical setting involves the Premier League and football clubs working with the Department of Health:

The Premier League and the Department of Health are developing plans to exploit football's popularity among men to help them overcome their notorious reluctance to visit a doctor, even when they are ill. Stadiums, famous for their meat pies and half-time cups of Bovril, will become places where fans are encouraged to seek treatment for obesity, heavy drinking or bowel cancer.

(Campbell 2004a: 7)

Ironically, the price of tickets at many premier clubs may mean that, although they may remain good venues to find men, these will not be among the most disadvantaged. According to Mark Bushell, curator of the National Football Museum: 'Football in the Premiership is becoming more and more gentrified. Certain tickets and certain types of seat clearly aren't aimed at traditional working class fans any more' (Campbell 2004b: 11).

These things matter because it can be all too easy to develop new services that will fail to address inequalities in access to health care. One illustration is a network of health centres targeted at busy commuters:

A network of walk-in health centres for commuters who find it difficult to consult their home GP during working hours was announced by the health secretary, John Reid, yesterday. He said the more customer-friendly NHS that Labour will promise at the next election will include walk-in centres in London, Newcastle, Leeds and Manchester where busy working people will be able to get immediate access to the full range of GP services.

(Carvel 2004: 10)

Developments of this type will undoubtedly address very real needs but may do nothing to improve equity in access. As has been shown, this is unlikely to be achieved without a deliberate and strategic intention to do so.

Creating the right level of state intervention

This brings us back to a question, originally raised very much earlier in the book, about the proper place for state intervention. Fears that professionals, acting on behalf of the state, become too closely involved in influencing and determining individual lifestyle choices need to be considered. So too do concerns that a less interventionist approach will merely allow inequalities in health between social groups to widen.

In part, responses to this will depend upon individual attitudes towards inequality and although the concept has formed a core theme through much of this book, it has not been possible to engage in some of the fundamental debates it has prompted in political and moral philosophy. However, there is one aspect that does need to be mentioned, relating to the comments by R.H. Tawney quoted at the beginning of this chapter.

Tawney urged the elimination of those inequalities having their source in the organization of society, and not those resulting from individual differences. Here it is relevant to recall studies described in Chapters 7, 8 and 9, particularly those which explored the relative contribution of lifestyle to health status. This played a significant role but no greater than many other factors. Robert Putnam concluded that the effect on health of not being involved in social groups was about the same as the damage done by smoking. The work of Michael Marmot and his colleagues suggested that less than one third of the social gradient in heart disease was attributable to risk factors including smoking.

Smoking causes immense damage to health and represents a genuine danger to public health that needs to be tackled. However, responses by governments and professionals can focus too easily upon aspects of individual behaviour without confronting the context in which it occurs. It is worth noting comments on this made in 1980 in the Black Report on health inequalities:

> Smoking is becoming more class-related. Tobacco and the tobacco industry are part of the material and cultural life of Britain – an important source of tax income for the government, still freely permitted in public places and backed up by a multi-million pound advertising campaign which includes sports sponsorship. This is changing, and there is a slow swing against smoking, but not surprisingly the avant garde of cultural change are drawn from the higher occupational classes. If cigarette smoking is a major contributory cause of deaths due to cancer or heart disease, then the uneven response in the population to the news that it is dangerous is likely, in future years, to make class differentials in health even wider than they are at present. This raises questions, of course, about the social and economic factors which explain the fact and the prevalence of smoking in the first place and whether these, independent of individual education or counselling, have to be given priority in reducing the differentials.
>
> (Townsend and Davidson 1982: 124)

One-quarter of a century later the prediction of widening class differentials in health has been born out, and yet a ban on smoking in public places was not included in a Government White Paper until the Autumn of 2004. Instead, the focus through much of the period has been upon changes in individual behaviour.

Smoking is an activity where personal and social influences intersect and interact but many other factors that contribute to poor health are even less amenable to individual control. Unemployment, long working hours, job stress and job control: all have been implicated as risks to good health. Yet constantly the spotlight is turned upon what the individual must do to avoid illness.

Unless professionals also address the wider determinants of health it seems to me that the charge of inappropriate intervention in personal behaviour could carry some weight. People should be supported in abandoning addictions to nicotine and encouraged not to delay seeking professional help when it is required. But much else is needed too.

Health inequalities will only be substantially reduced with a simultaneous attack upon the causes of poor health and an improvement in early interventions for those most at risk. Health professionals have a potentially important role to play in this but caution must be exercised in how this develops. For example, a proposal by the Chancellor of the Exchequer to find new ways of encouraging claimants of incapacity benefit into work have met doubts from some quarters:

> Doctors have expressed concern at proposals to introduce Job Centre staff into GP surgeries as part of the government's effort to combat what it has called Britain's burgeoning 'sick note culture'. A spokesman for the British Medical Association said: 'Doctors are not there to help police the social security system ... We would have concern if patients were put under stress by the presence of an employment adviser at their surgery. The focus should be on getting fit people back to work.'
>
> The chancellor's report said advisers will be installed in surgeries as part of a focus on 'fitness for work advice' for patients with health conditions they think might impact their ability to work. Government advice on combating the 'sick note culture' will also be extended to doctors themselves, who are to have their 'awareness of the implications of sickness absence improved'. Employment advisers, said a spokesman for the department of work and pensions, are to be 'part of the surgery team'.
>
> *(Guardian* 03.12.04)

Fears may be misplaced, as this could provide an example of the type of wider support that has been discussed previously. It should also be noted that, as has earlier been described, one of the largest groups of claimants receiving Incapacity Benefit are those with mental illness. Survey evidence indicates that these are also the most likely to be wanting work: 86 per cent compared to 52 per cent for all disabled people (cited in TUC 2004: 5). Attention must also be given to the stigma that may make gaining employment difficult and how this is to be addressed.

Other ways of addressing these issues might prove more successful. For many health professionals, this is likely to require working in new ways. For example, trade unions could be important partners in addressing occupational health issues. Advice agencies have vital experiences in dealing with the type of problems that for far too many people are soul-destroying and debilitating. Community associations and tenants' groups can offer opportunities to engage with people who might not become involved in NHS-centred initiatives. The list could go on but the need is to identify ways of addressing the causes of ill-health over which people feel they have little control. This should not be another opportunity to exert the control of the professional but to support people taking greater control themselves. This could provide a firm foundation for a model of health care based upon choice, a theme addressed in the concluding section of this book.

Conclusion
Choice, trust and responsibility

Patient choice figures prominently in many debates about the health service. It represents a response to evidence that individuals want greater control over what they receive as consumers. It is a trend that is not unique to health care.

However, there is another rationale for backing choice. This is the argument, advanced by economists such as Frederick Hayek, that experts cannot possibly know what people really want. It is claimed that only inefficiency will result if too much attempt is made to plan things. Markets must be allowed to operate and although some will fail in the marketplace, the more efficient will prosper. Benefits will spread, but for markets to function in this way individuals must be able to make their own choices. To restrict this is not only an unwarranted paternalism but inefficient with it.

These two arguments in favour of choice can appear symmetrical; while one stresses the benefits of choice for individuals, the other does so for society. Everyone is better off. And this is how they often are presented, as mutually supportive arguments, justifying the same conclusion.

Up to a point they do. But the argument for choice based on it producing an efficient allocation of resources makes no assumption about the quality of each individual choice. This can be illustrated by a couple of examples. The first dates from 1906, when the statistician Sir Francis Galton observed visitors at a livestock show enter a competition to guess the weight of an ox. There were 800 entries and the mean of the 800 guesses was 1197 pounds. This average was only one pound less than the actual weight of the ox. It is almost uncanny, but of course many guesses were wide off the mark. These, in effect, cancelled each other out. For each person who underestimated there was someone who overestimated.

A similar example comes from the sinking of a US submarine, *Scorpion*, in the north Atlantic in 1968. A disparate group of people estimated where the submarine had sunk and she was found just 2202 yards from the mid-point of the different estimates. No one estimate had actually come as close as this average (Surowiecki 2004).

Giving people choices may produce a good optimum result but many may get the answer wrong. A basic dilemma for professional work is how to assist in overcoming these errors while avoiding the paternalism of the past. Central to this is the notion of trust. A significant minority of parents today may show a lack of trust in scientific opinion on matters such as the MMR vaccine, but we can put this into perspective. It pales into insignificance in comparison to past controversies over vaccination.

When the vaccination of infants against smallpox was made compulsory in the nineteenth century, it generated substantial opposition, although there were considerable variations. In Leicester, at the heart of the protest, 6000 people were prosecuted in a 20-year period and at one time two-thirds of the local police were required to keep order as goods seized to pay fines were auctioned. A demonstration in 1885 drew 20,000 people. The campaign in Leicester had its effect, as rates of vaccination fell from 60 per cent in the early 1880s to a mere 4 per cent by 1889 (Baldwin 1999). It was not until 1898 that a clause was introduced allowing exceptions if parents could convince two magistrates that they held conscientious objections. From 1907, all that was required was a statement of objection and the proportion of vaccinated infants declined from 78 per cent in 1906 to barely 60 per cent in 1909. Compulsion was removed entirely with the establishment of the NHS, with the rate eventually falling to 27 per cent, until routine vaccination was discontinued in the 1970s as the disease was vanquished (Baldwin, 1999: 302).

Although not on the same scale, there are also notable variations in rates of uptake of the MMR vaccine. Local immunization data shows that the take-up in Dorset and Berkshire, for instance, fell by eight percentage points from 1998–9 to 2001–2 (to 82 per cent and 74 per cent, respectively). In contrast, Barnsley saw rates drop by just one percentage point during the same period: but this only took it to 93 per cent, a rate higher than the national average had been in 1998. To use one further example, no decline at all occurred in Salford and Trafford, where the rate remained at 90 per cent (NHS Immunisation Statistics for England: 1998–9 and 2001–2).

This suggests complex processes, with many factors contributing to local characteristics. To engage successfully with these, professionals must not only gain an understanding of them but also develop styles of interaction with patients that allow alternative views to be expressed and discussed. Not all current proposals seem to be moving in this direction.

Contracts for health care?

'Fat people will have to diet if they want to see the doctor', warned *The Times* on 3 June 2003, announcing a story about Labour's new policy paper on Health and Social Care. This included a proposed new 'agreement' between patients and their GPs of which a 'senior Health Department source' is quoted as saying: 'This document is about kick-starting the debate. As the NHS gets better, the issue of the patient's responsibilities becomes more stark.'

The next day a Labour Party spokesperson told *The Independent* newspaper: 'This is a serious political debate about how we change the relationship between public services and individual members of the public to one where people understand the rights we enjoy depend on the duties we owe.'

By this time others were entering the debate – Dr John Chisholm, the chairman of the British Medical Association general practitioners committeee, told *The*

Daily Telegraph: 'The proposals seem to threaten the doctor–patient relationship and potentially seem even to deny people the free care to which I believe they are entitled.'

The Labour Party document that provoked the controversy explained that 'this type of agreement would not be legally binding' but added that it could: 'bind the patient into honouring their duty to the health service, putting the relationship onto a statutory footing'.

The centrality of patient duty and responsibility is indicated in comments anticipating opposition: 'To win support for this we need to be clear about what it is that we are trying to do – we must emphasise that in return for free, convenient, high quality care the patient is being asked to use this resource responsibly.'

Once more, the focus is upon the responsibility of the individual. Contracts can imply a perceived low level of trust. Even though not regarded as legally binding, they are a means of defining and making formal the reciprocal duties in a relationship. This has potential implications for levels of trust between professionals and patients. A recent report by the Audit Commission (2003), based on data provided by MORI, suggests relatively little change in levels of trust shown towards individual occupational groups. The group most highly trusted, by 91 per cent of respondents, was doctors, compared to 18 per cent who trusted politicans.

Trust in professional groups tended to be higher than in institutions – for instance, only 71 per cent said they would trust the NHS. As one member of a MORI focus group commented: 'You trust individuals rather than the organisation they represent. So you trust doctors and nurses, for example, but you wouldn't trust the NHS as a whole.'

Some institutions fared even worse. Only 22 per cent said they trusted 'big companies'. Many people regarded the public sector as less efficient but placed higher levels of trust in it. In the words of one person: 'Ultimately public services are there for the public, no matter how inefficient they are. It is almost an impossible job for them. Private is not about equality, it's about personal gain.'

It is relevant here to note a distinction between primary and secondary trust. Primary trust refers to 'the estimate of the trustworthiness of the target on which we are considering whether to confer trust' (Sztompka 1999: 70–1), but as this can require considerable information and familiarity, secondary trust involves institutional arrangements that are assumed to guarantee trustworthiness: 'Accountability means the enforcement of trustworthiness, or more precisely the presence of agencies monitoring and sanctioning the conduct of the trustee, or at least potentially available for such monitoring and sanctioning if the breach of trust occurs' (Sztompka 1999: 87).

Most public trust in professionals is largely based on this, in the belief that the professions are adequately monitored and regulated. Nevertheless, there is evidence that levels of trust are declining. As the point of contact between the patient and the state, the role of the professional is subject to competing demands. For instance, a controversial issue for many publicly provided health care systems in recent years has been whether a fully comprehensive range of services should be available. Rationing of some kind has always existed. Waiting lists are intended as a means of ordering provision to ensure that those individuals with the greatest clinical need receive attention before those with a lesser need. Other kinds of rationing have simply removed discrete areas of treatment. By 1996, for example, almost 70 treatments had been withdrawn by at least one health authority in England and Wales, including in vitro fertilization, reversal of male vasectomy and female sterilization, the removal of tattoos and sex change operations (Butler 1999: 21).

Many professionals work within state organizations but, at the same time, must demonstrate a measure of independence from them. Without this, levels of trust are likely to continue downwards. Public scepticism towards authority of many kinds may sometimes be judged unfair or wrong, but is rarely entirely groundless. It was not so many years ago that the link between tobacco and lung cancer was contested, with the Health Minister telling Parliament in the 1950s that public warnings should not be issued because presence of a carcinogenic substance in tobacco was not yet certain (Cartwright 1983: 27).

Much more is now known of how tobacco companies have subsequently operated. Documents obtained from Phillip Morris (one of the world's largest tobacco companies, producing top-selling brands such as Malboro and Chester-field) and placed on a website exposing the advertising tactics of the tobacco companies reveal:

Our objective remains to develop and mobilize the necessary resources – internal Philip Morris, external agencies and consultants, the industry National Marketing Associations, and all potential allies – to fight the social and legislative initiatives against tobacco ... We shall carefully target our opponents. We shall precisely identify, monitor, isolate, and contest key individuals and organizations.
(Philip Morris 1989 quoted in Hammond and Rowell 2001)

Explaining a strategy designed to shape the way in which debate on tobacco products develops, another internal document states the aim as being to: 'Portray the debate as one between the anti-tobacco lobby and the smoker, instead of "pro-health public citizens" versus the tobacco industry' (Philip Morris 1992 quoted in Hammond and Rowell 2001).

Mindful of this type of behaviour, many people are anxious about how decisions are made, who makes them and in whose interests. This can also create a basis for challenges to powerful organizations judged to be acting in a self-interested manner. In the controversy over the antidepressant, Seroxat, a report in *The Observer* describes how new forms of electronic communication may be facilitating opportunities for collective responses. GlaxoSmithKline (GSK) denied that Seroxat was responsible for causing any harm to children for whom it had been prescribed, but nevertheless agreed to settle a $2.5 million lawsuit in New York, in which it was accused of fraud for concealing evidence about the drug:

> The GSK suit created the tipping point in the pharmas' change of fortune and has revealed the force behind it. The formal complaint drew heavily on research by public health campaigners and consumer advocates about the hazards of anti-depressant use. These activists had toiled in deepest obscurity – some of them, for a decade – until their discoveries were featured on a Panorama programme, 'Secrets of Seroxat', in autumn 2002. A follow-up broadcast the next spring, 'Emails from the edge', analysed 1,370 messages from viewers about the first programme, mostly from people reporting antidepressant withdrawal reaction including shock-like sensations in their heads, and thoughts about self-mutilation, violence and suicide.
>
> (*The Observer* 29.09.04)

The journalist comments that bodies such as the Royal College of Psychiatrists had endorsed the safety of the drug, prior to GSK eventually amending the prescribing guidelines. She argues that:

> The events that led to Seroxat's exposure would seem to suggest that it was television power that forced GSK to recant. But it was really the internet that allowed public health activists to do an end run around GSK's and the medical authorities' denials of the drug's risks. An explosion of websites dedicated to vivid accounts of anti-depressant reactions told these campaigners about hundreds of thousands affected by a problem that officially did not exist.
>
> (*The Observer* 29.09.04)

Responsibility lies at the heart of the relationship between choice and trust. We all want to exercise more choice but sometimes we need expert guidance. Objecting to paternalism does not require dismissing the value of expertise. It takes different forms and professionals must acknowledge this as much as their critics. Individuals have responsibilities but are not alone in this. A responsibility of professionals is to apply judgement and expertise in a manner that acknowledges each person's individuality and autonomy while understanding the social constraints within which this is exercised. Individual choice requires that the social barriers to its effective development are better understood and more firmly challenged.

Appendix: Marx, Weber and Durkheim

The ideas of several social theorists from the mid-nineteenth to early twentieth century are introduced in this book, which may puzzle some readers who are looking for ideas to help understand health care developments in today's Britain. There is a straightforward explanation. These writers, often known as classical social theorists, were interested in trying to understand and explain the processes of social change and modernization occurring in their own time. The context of today is very different but if we are prepared to expend a little effort acquainting ourselves with the underlying concepts, the ideas of these writers provide important insights that have continuing relevance.

More recent theorists, including those sometimes described as postmodernists, do not feature to the same extent in this book. This would have taken it in a rather different direction, but in any event their ideas are best understood in the context of the contribution of classical social theory.

For readers for whom these ideas may be unfamiliar, the following provides a short introduction to three of the most prominent figures: Karl Marx, Max Weber and Emil Durkheim. The book, *Classical Social Theory*, by Ian Craib (1997), is one to which readers who seek a fuller account of these theorists are encouraged to turn.

Karl Marx (1818–83)

Karl Marx was born in Trier, in the German Rhineland, in 1818. The son of a lawyer (a Jew who converted to Christianity following the introduction of anti-Jewish laws in 1816), Marx embarked on what looked to be a successful academic career. After studying law in Berlin he went on to complete a doctorate in philosophy, although while in Berlin he was attracted to the company of politically radical thinkers. Despite his proven academic ability, this threatened his prospects of gaining an academic post, causing him to turn instead to radical journalism.

The first paper on which he worked was soon closed down by the authorities. It had published an article attacking the authoritarianism of the Russian political system, and Marx was forced to leave Germany. He married and moved to Paris in 1843, where he embarked upon a detailed analysis of German philosophy and British economists. His time in Paris was short but important: the way Marx uses the concept of alienation, discussed in Chapter 9, was developed in his *Economic and Philosophical Manuscripts* during this time. Paris also brought him into contact with French socialism, a crucial influence on his emerging ideas. However, he came to the attention of the French authorities and was expelled from the country in 1845.

Moving to Brussels, Marx began what became a lifelong collaboration with Frederich Engels. In 1848 they jointly wrote and published the *Communist Manifesto*, a statement of their political thinking. This was a time of enormous political upheaval, with radical and revolutionary movements challenging the power of established regimes across Europe. Inevitably, Marx was expelled from Brussels and after moving back to Germany was once again forced to flee. The one country in Europe prepared to accept him was Britain, where Marx spent the main part of his adult life in exile, from 1849 until his death in 1883.

It was in London that much of his writing was done, including his major work of political economy, *Capital*. Marx emphasized the importance of economic relationships for understanding how societies function. He did not believe, as is sometimes suggested, that economic relationships determined everything but he started from the view that the economic base of society (for example, whether this was feudal or capitalist) was a fundamental determinant of the character of social relationships within it. He also acknowledged the constraints within which human activity occurs, as in these remarks in his 1852 analysis of Louis Napoleon's seizure of power in France the previous year:

> Men make their own history, but they do not make it just as they please; they do not make it under circumstances chosen by themselves, but under circumstances directly encountered, given and transmitted from the past. The tradition of all the dead generations weighs like a nightmare on the minds of the living.
>
> (Marx 1978: 9)

Marx believed that as capitalism had challenged and superseded feudal relationships by creating a new, working class, it brought into being a social force that would eventually cause its overthrow. Because of the links Marx made between his social analysis and political objectives, he became an influential source for twentieth-century political movements seeking to achieve those aims. One consequence has been his association in the minds of some with Stalinist totalitarian regimes, a link that even the most cursory reading of his work shows to be baseless.

Marx's goal was human emancipation and he paid particular attention to arguing that work should be inherently fulfilling, and not simply engaged in as a means to an end. He saw work under capitalism as alienating (described in Chapter 9) and regarded the reduction of the working day as a priority. For this to be achieved, he argued, it would be necessary to replace the unpredictable workings of the market with a more rational system:

> Freedom in this field can only consist in socialised man, the associated producers, rationally regulating their interchange with Nature, bringing it under

their common control, instead of being ruled by it as by the blind forces of Nature.

(Marx quoted in Wolff 2002: 97)

Marx's vision of a new society was not of monochrome equality but an allocation of resources that matched people's needs. As he wrote in 1875, in the communism he envisaged, society would: 'inscribe on its banner: from each according to his ability; to each according to his need' (Marx quoted in Wolff 2002: 95).

Some may dismiss this as hopeless utopianism, although the principle is reflected in the underlying philosophy of the National Health Service. Marx, however, tended to concentrate on analysing capitalism rather than describing what might replace it. An important strand in his thinking was that social change required the active participation of the working class and could not be left to experts.

From his analysis of capitalism, two particular concepts deserve attention, each related to what he regarded as the central aspect of human activity: labour. The two concepts are alienation and exploitation.

A brief account of alienation is provided in Chapter 9 and need not be repeated here. Marx saw labour under capitalism as being treated as a commodity, bought and sold like other goods. It was the dehumanizing consequences that Marx highlighted, arguing that this worsened as more and more commodities were produced. As he describes it in his 1844 Manuscripts, in a message possessing continuing resonance today: 'With the increasing value of the world of things proceeds in direct proportion the devaluation of the world of men' (Marx 1974: 107).

The concept of exploitation is used by Marx to describe the economic relationship between workers and capitalists. It does not refer to oppression, which may arise in many contexts, but to what Marx regarded as a fundamental feature of capitalism: that the value of what workers produce is more than they receive in wages and salaries. This extra value (or surplus value) represents the exploitation of workers, and in Marx's view, intensifies as capitalism develops.

His description of attempts to lengthen the working day, also referred to in Chapter 9, provide an example.

Marx gave little direct attention to issues of health and illness. However, his use of the concepts of alienation and exploitation provide valuable guides for thinking about human experiences in the context of modern, global capitalism. The sources of these may be more geographically distant but they remain nonetheless real.

Marx was a powerful and original social thinker, and an important aspect of his character retains current relevance. This was his view that theory always had a purpose and that its relationship with practice must constantly be tested. On his tombstone in Highgate Cemetery are words taken from a piece he wrote in response to the German philosopher, Ludwig Feurbach: 'The philosophers have only interpreted the world in various ways; the point is to change it.'

Max Weber (1864–1920)

Born nearly half a century after Marx, Max Weber was brought up in Berlin, where Marx had been a student. Weber's father was a lawyer who went on to become a senior government official and the milieu in which the young Weber grew up was one of professional, academic and political discussion. He too embarked upon the study of law, entering the University of Heidelberg in 1882. Again like Marx, he was fond of drinking, carousing and duelling. Unlike Marx, Weber went on to pursue a formal academic career.

Gaining a professorship in political economy at the University of Freiberg, he went on to be appointed Professor of Economics at the University of Heidelberg in 1896. However, this progress was checked in the following year, following the death of his father. The death occurred shortly after an argument between the two men and had an immediate impact on Weber's emotional state. In 1898, after several years of intense work, and at the very point when his career was flourishing, Max Weber suffered a nervous breakdown.

Weber found the pressure of academic work impossible to maintain and instead he embarked upon a period of travelling; across Europe and (in 1904) to the US. Returning from the US he completed his book, *The Protestant Ethic and the Spirit of Capitalism*. Weber had long been interested in religion, distinguishing what he saw as an important difference between dominant Western and Eastern belief systems. This related to Judaism's emphasis on the notion of a chosen people, the Children of God, who would have their proper place restored. In Weber's words: 'The whole attitude toward life of ancient Jewry was determined by this conception of a future God-oriented political and social revolution' (Weber 1952: 5).

The Old Testament prophets articulate this conception, representing a tradition of ethically-guided behaviour designed to improve the world. This ethical dimension, emphasizing the values upon which social action proceeds, provides for Weber an important means of explaining social change; including the emergence of capitalism and modernity. Weber argued that a new ethic arose, giving encouragement to 'the earning of more and more money ... Man is dominated by the making of money, by acquisition as the ultimate purpose of his life' (Weber 1930: 53).

Weber acknowledged the role played by the pursuit of material interests, which is dominant in Marx's account, but he asked why, in the Europe of his day, many business leaders and owners of capital, as well as many skilled and technical workers, were Protestant (Weber 1930: 35). His answer lay in the argument that Protestantism, particularly Calvinism, encouraged a disciplined approach to work as a duty. He was not suggesting this 'caused' capitalism but rather tracing the connections between religion and aspects of the culture of early capitalism.

This is an example of one of Weber's key contributions to sociological thinking: to point to the role of subjective intention. As he remarks:

> While statistical correlations may sensitize us to the possibility of a causal link, such a link can only be established if we satisfy ourselves that there is a connecting sequence of motivation.

> (Weber, cited in Parkin 2002: 21)

Following the publication of *The Protestant Ethic* in 1904, Weber's prodigious output resumed until, with the outbreak of war in 1914, he was put in charge of administration in his local hospital. It seems he wanted to enlist, but at 50 was too old. By the later part of the war he returned to scholarship, much of which provides the source for his account of rationalization in modern society. Weber's work on religion is important for understanding his ideas about rationality, a short summary of which is provided in Chapters 2 and 3 of this book. Here it is only necessary to develop one aspect.

This concerns methods by which authority and domination are exercised, summarized by Weber in three forms: charismatic, traditional and legal-rational. The first refers to the role of individual personality in leadership, while the second describes the acceptance of arrangements based on custom. Weber saw these being replaced in the modern state by legal-rational domination, in which the legitimacy of power rests upon its being exercised rationally. This required officials and experts to act in accordance with rules, calculating the merits of action on evidence rather than sectional interest. It was a system of authority he described as 'bureaucratic'.

Max Weber died in 1920, at the age of 56, and much of his writing on these themes was published posthumously. In one such piece of work he points to sources of conflict that can arise between bureaucracy and democracy:

> Once it is fully established, bureaucracy is among those social structures which are among the hardest to destroy ... and where the bureaucratization of administration has been completely carried through, a form of power relation is established that is practically unshatterable ... After all, bureaucracy strives merely to level those powers that stand in its way and in those areas that, in the individual case, it seeks to occupy. We must remember this fact – which we have encountered several times and which we shall have to discuss repeatedly: that 'democracy' as such is opposed to the rule of 'bureaucracy'.
>
> (Weber, cited in Lee and Newby 1983: 193)

Weber was a liberal and towards the end of his life unsuccessfully sought nomination as a candidate for the newly-founded German Democratic Party. His sociology was based on a view that emphasized the individual meaning of actions; that people face choices and these are not determined by inevitable forces. He was also aware of what he described as the 'iron cage' of bureaucracy, a feature that requires constant vigilance if excessive domination is to be avoided. Subsequent developments in technology and expertise make this issue just as relevant today, particularly in the context of how we deal with health, illness and suffering. Weber reminds us of the importance of considering the values on which these choices are made.

Emil Durkheim (1858–1917)

Durkheim was born in France in 1858, the son of a long line of Jewish rabbis. Like Weber, Emil Durkheim pursued a relatively formal academic career. Although, as a student in Paris, he showed support for liberal and democratic reforms in opposition to right-wing monarchists, he remained aloof from political activity.

Following his graduation, Durkheim taught philosophy before travelling to Germany where he encountered new developments in psychology and social science. He was considerably interested in the approach he observed there towards scientific method, which influenced his thinking when he returned to take up the first social science post at a French University, in Bordeaux, in 1887.

In his book, *Rules of Sociological Method*, published in 1895, Durkheim describes what he calls 'social facts', by which he referred to factors that were external to individuals and constrained their behaviour. As an illustration, the legal acceptance of tobacco and prohibition of marijuana as a 'social fact' reveals a contrast in social acceptability and tradition, rather than any other consideration. Durkheim also discusses the relationship between the normal and the pathological, drawing on a biological analogy to offer important insights into how these emerge as social categories.

An enduring theme running through Durkheim's work is the consequences of different types of social organization for the psychological and emotional experiences of individuals. This is illustrated in his books, *The Division of Labour*, published in 1893 and *Suicide*, published in 1896. Both are referred to in Chapter 8 in a discussion on society, relationships and health.

Durkheim continually emphasized the importance of social factors for individuals. In discussions on the development of knowledge, for instance, he argued that the mind works with categories that are initially social in their origin. He used the term 'collective consciousness' to refer to these socially-established categories of thinking. This focus has encouraged many to judge Durkheim as a conservative thinker, a view given support by comments such as these on morality: 'it is never possible to desire a morality other than that required by the social conditions of a given time' (Durkheim, quoted in Craib 1997: 76).

However, Durkheim was also aware of the need for social change, although he rejected revolutionary action. He described himself as a socialist, although his was the socialism of administrative expertise and efficiency rather than popular participation and the labour movement. Although he gave primacy to the role of social factors when explaining individual behaviour, as in his analysis of suicide, he believed strongly in the importance of the individual and individual rights.

This is illustrated in Durkheim's only involvement in politics, which came about as a consequence of the Dreyfus case. This originated from fears within the French army that secret information was being given to the Germans. Suspicion fell on a captain, Alfred Dreyfus. He had access to the information involved and he was also a Jew, and despite his claims of innocence was found guilty of treason by court martial and sentenced to life imprisonment on Devil's Island. The conviction of Dreyfus intensified the vilification of Jews in sections of the press.

Few were prepared to stand by him, with the most notable exception being the novelist, Emile Zola. Zola's attack on the decision, published under the title *J'accuse!*, led to him being found guilty of libel. Another who spoke out was Durkheim but it took 12 years for the miscarriage of justice to be acknowledged and Dreyfus could return to Paris to have his former rank restored.

Observing the public response to the conviction of Dreyfus, Durkheim gives a crushing indictment of those who seek scapegoats for society's ills:

When society undergoes suffering, it feels the need to find someone whom it can hold responsible for its sickness, on whom it can avenge its misfortunes: and those against whom public opinion already discriminates are naturally designated for this role. These are the pariahs who serve as expiatory victims. What confirms me in this interpretation is the way in which the result of Dreyfus's trial was greeted in 1894. There was a surge of joy on the boulevards. People celebrated as a triumph what should have been a cause for public mourning. At last they knew whom to blame for the economic troubles and moral distress in which they lived. The trouble came from the Jews. The charge had been officially proved. By this very fact alone, things already seemed to be getting better and people felt consoled.

(Quoted in Lukes 1992: 345)

Durkheim continued his academic work after the Dreyfus case, taking the view that academics have a responsibility to take a stand on major political issues but not to embark upon the role of politician or statesman.

The First World War brought personal tragedy to Durkheim's family, as to millions of others. His son, Andre, was reported missing during the French retreat from Serbia in early 1916. The impact on Durkheim was immense; his work immediately declined and later that year he suffered a stroke. Despite showing some signs of recovery during the following spring, Durkheim died in the summer of 1917, aged 59.

His work later gained renewed influence through the American sociologist, Talcott Parsons, who perhaps tended to reinforce the conservative image of him. It is more accurate to regard him as someone who sought to understand individual behaviour as social behaviour but without losing sight of the need to retain a profound sense of individual responsibility. There are many contexts today in which Durkheim's refusal to succumb to popular emotions offers a powerful and relevant example. Too many politicians and media seem prepared to stoke public anxieties about patients with mental illness living in the community; asylum seekers with substantial health care needs find themselves a target of vilification and abuse; and it is becoming increasingly common for victims of illness to find themselves unreasonably accused of responsibility for their condition. With illness, and factors associated with it, providing a significant opportunity for creating scapegoats, we should heed Durkheim's call, made in the context of the Dreyfus case, for people to: 'have the courage to proclaim aloud what they think, and to unite together in order to achieve victory in the struggle against public madness' (quoted in Lukes 1992: 347).

References

Abel-Smith, B. and Townsend, P. (1965) *The Poor and the Poorest*. Bell, London.

Abercrombie, N., Hall, S. and Turner, B. (1984) *Penguin Dictionary of Sociology*. Penguin, Harmondsworth.

Albrow, M. (1970) *Bureaucracy*. Macmillan, London.

Allsop, J. (1984) *Health Policy and the National Health Service*. Longman.

Allsop, J. (1995) *Health Policy and the NHS: Towards 2000*. Longman, London.

American Academy of Pediatrics (2001) 'Measles-mumps-rubella vaccine and autistic spectrum disorder: A report from the new challenges in childhood immunisation conference'. www.aap.org/advocacy/archives/mayautmmr.htm.

Arie, S. and Burke, J. (2004) 'Who Cares?' *The Observer*, 15 August.

Arksey, M. (1994) 'Expert and lay participation in the construction of medical knowledge', *Sociology of Health and Illness*. 16(4): 448–68.

Asthana, S. *et al*. 'Inequalities in Health Service Utilisation at the General Practice Level'. Economic and Social Research Council Summary report.

Audit Commission/MORI Social Research Institute (2003) *Exploring Trust in Public Institutions*. MORI Social Research Institute.

Bain, G.S. and Price, R. (1983) 'Union Growth: Dimensions, Determinants and Destiny' in G.S. Bain (ed.) *Industrial Relations in Britain*. Basil Blackwell, Oxford.

Baldwin, P. (1999) *Contagion and the State in Europe, 1830–1930*. Cambridge University Press, Cambridge.

Balint, M. (1957) *The Doctor, his Patient and the Illness*. Pitman, London. Cited in Tuckett and Kaufert (1978): 135–8.

Barham, C. and Leonard, J. (2002) 'Trends and sources of data on sickness', *Labour Market Trends*, April 2002: 177–85.

Barnes, B. (1995) *The Elements of Social Theory*. UCL Press, London.

Barrett, J.F., Jarvis, G.J., MacDonald, H.N., Bucham, P.C., Tyrrell, S.N. and Lilford, R.J. (1990) 'Inconsistencies in clinical decisions in obstetrics' *The Lancet* 336: 549–51.

Bartley, M., Sacker, A. and Clarke, P. (2004) 'Employment status, employment conditions, and limiting illness: prospective evidence from the British household panel survey 1991–2001', *Journal of Epidemiology and Community Health* 58: 501–6.

BBC (2002) Newsnight: Why don't parents believe MMR is safe? Broadcast 6 February. Transcript on www.news.bbc.co.uk/1/hi/events/newsnight/1807646.stm.

BBC (2003) *Panorama – Seroxat: e-mails from the edge*. Transmitted 11th May 2003.

Beck, U. (1992) *Risk Society: Towards a New Modernity*. Sage, London.

Beckman, H.B. and Frankel, R.M (1984) 'The effect of physician behaviour on the collection of data', *Annals of Internal Medicine* 101: 692–6.

Bell, D. (1974) *The Coming of Post-Industrial Society: a venture in social forecasting*. Heinemann Educational, London.

Ben-Shlomo, Y. and Chaturvedi, N. (1995) 'Assessing equity in access to health care provision in the UK: does where you live affect your chances of getting a coronary bypass graft?', *Journal of Epidemiology and Community Health* 49: 200–4.

Benzeval, M. and Donald, A. (1999) 'The role of the NHS in tackling inequalities in health', in D. Gordon, M. Shaw, D. Dorling and G. Davey (eds) *Inequalities in Health: the evidence presented to the Independent Inquiry into Inequalities in Health, Chaired by Sir Donald Acheson*. Policy Press, Bristol.

Berger, P. and Luckmann, T. (1971) (originally 1966) *The Social Construction of Reality: a treatise in the sociology of knowledge*. Penguin, Harmondsworth.

Blair, T. (1995) The Spectator/Allied Dunbar lecture, *The Spectator*, 25 March.

Blair, T. (2002) 'New Labour and Community', *Renewal: A Journal of Labour politics* 10 (2).

Blair, T. (2003) Speech at the South Camden Community College, London. www.labour.org.uk/news/tbsocialjustice.

Blatchford, O., Capewell, S., Mirray, S. and Blatchford, M. (1999) 'Emergency medical admission in Glasgow: general practices vary despite adjustments for age, sex and deprivation', *British Journal of Medical Practice* 19: 551–4.

Blaxter, M. (1983) 'The Cause of Disease', Women Talking *Social Science and Medicine* 17 (2): 59–69.

Blaxter, M. (1990) *Health and Lifestyles*. Tavistock/Routledge, London.

Blofield, Sir John (2003) *Independent Inquiry into the death of David Bennett*. Presented to the Secretary of State for Health and the Norfolk, Suffolk and Cambridgeshire Strategic Health Authority, December 2003.

Bobbio, N. (1996) *Left and Right: The Significance of a Political Distinction*. Polity Press/Blackwell Publishers

Bocock, R. and Thompson, K. (1992) *Social and Cultural Forms of Modernity*. Open University Press/Polity Press.

Bodenheimer, T.S. (1984) 'The transnational pharmaceutical industry and the health of the world's people' in J.B. McKinlay (ed.) *Issues in the Political Economy of Health Care*. Tavistock Publications.

Bonaccorso, S.N. and Sturchio J.L. (2002) 'Education and debate: Direct to consumer advertising is medicalising normal human experience: Against', *British Medical Journal* 324: 910–11.

Bosma, H., Marmot, M., Hemingway, H., Nicholson, A., Brunner, E. and Stansfeld, S. (1997) 'Low job control and risk of coronary heart disease in Whitehall II (prospective cohort) study', *British Medical Journal* 314: 558.

Boswell, D. (1992) 'Health, the Self and Social Interaction', in R. Bocock and K. Thompson *Social and Cultural Forms of Modernity*. Open University Press/Polity Press.

Bott, E. (1957) *Family and Social Network*. Tavistock, London.

Bottomore, T. and Rubel, M. (1963) *Karl Marx: Selected Writings in Sociology and Social Philosophy*. Penguin, Harmondsworth.

Brewin, T. (1995) 'Truth, trust and paternalism' in B. Davey, A. Gray and C. Seale, *Health and Disease: A Reader* (2nd edition). Open University Press, Buckingham.

Briggs, A. (1961) 'Cholera and Society in the Nineteenth Century Past and Present', *A Journal of Historical Studies* 19: 76–96.

British Medical Association (1986) *Alternative Therapy*. BMA, London.

British Medical Journal (1948) 'Streptomycin treatment of pulmonary tuberculosis: a Medical Research Council investigation' (ii: 769–82 October 30).

British Medical Journal (1999) 'Editorial: Paternalism or Partnership', *British Medical Journal* 319: 719–20.

Britten, N. (1991) 'Hospital consultants' views of their patients', *Sociology of Health and Illness* 13 (1): 83–97.

Brown, J.A.C. (1954) *The Social Psychology of Industry*. Penguin, Harmondsworth.

Brown, P. (1995) 'Popular epidemiology, toxic waste and social movements', in J. Gabe (ed.) *Medicine, Health and Risk: Sociological Approaches*. Blackwell Publishers.

Brown, T. and Harris, G. (1979) *Social Origins of Depression: A Study of Psychiatric Disorder in Women*. Tavistock Publications.

Bruhn, J.G. and Wolf, S. (1979) *The Roseto Story*. University of Oklahoma Press, Norman, OK.

Brunner, E. (1997) 'Socioeconomic determinants of health: stress and the biology of inequality', *British Medical Journal*, 314: 1472–76.

Bunker J.P. (2001) 'Medicine Matters After All', in B. Davey, A. Gray and C. Seale *Health and Disease: A Reader* (3rd edition). Open University Press, Buckingham.

Burchfield, R.W. (1996) *The New Fowler's Modern English Usage*. Oxford University Press, Oxford.

Burns, T. (ed.) (1969) *Industrial Man: Selected Readings*. Penguin, Harmondsworth.

Butler, J. (1999) *The Ethics of Health Care Rationing: Principles and Practice*. Cassell, London.

Butler, S. (1970) *Erewhon*. Penguin Classics.

Butterworth, E. and Weir, D. (eds) (1976) *The Sociology of Modern Britain* (revised edition). Fontana/Collins.

Calman, K. and Hine, D. (1995) *A Policy Framework for Commissioning Cancer*. Department of Health, London.

Cameron, A. (1996) in N. Bobbio *Left and Right: The Significance of a Political Distinction*. Polity Press/Blackwell Publishers.

Campbell Semple, J. (1991) 'Tenosynovitis, repetitive strain injury, cumulative trauma disorder, and overuse syndrome, et cetera', *The Journal of Bone and Joint Surgery* 73 (4): 536–8.

Campbell, D. (2004a) 'Football fans to get physicals as clubs seek a clinical finish', *The Observer* 19.9.04, p. 7.

Campbell, D. (2004b) 'Super seats set new world record for watching football', *The Observer* 28.11.04, p.11.

Cartwright, A. (1983) *Health Surveys in practice and potential*. King's Fund, London.

Cartwright, A. and Marshall, J. (1965) *Medical Care* 3: 69.

Cartwright, A. and O'Brien, M (1976) 'Social class variations in health care and in the nature of GP consultations', *Sociological Review*, Monograph 22. University of Keele.

Carvel, J. (2004) 'Commuters to get GP centres in big cities', *Guardian*, 30.9.04, p. 10.

Castells, M. (1996) *The Information Age Vol 1: The Rise of the Network Society*. Blackwell.

Clark, J.M. (1981) 'Communication in Nursing': *Nursing Times* 1.1.81, 12–18.

Cohen, S., Doyle, W.J., Skoner, D.P., Rabin, B.S. and Gwaltney, J.M. (1997) 'Social ties and susceptibility to the common cold', *Journal of the American Medical Association* 277: 1940–4.

Coleman, D. (2000) 'Population and family' in A.H. Halsey and J. Webb (eds) *Twentieth Century British Social Trends*. Macmillan, London.

Collins, M. (2003) *Modern Love: An Intimate History of Men and Women in Twentieth-Century Britain*. Atlantic Books, London.

Cooper, L. (1997) 'Myalgic Encephalomyelitis and the medical encounter', *Sociology of Health and Illness* 19 (2): 186–207.

Cooper, M.H. and Culyer, A.J. (1972) 'Equality in the National Health Service. Intentions, performance and problems in evaluation', in M.M. Hauser (cd.) *The Economics of Medical Care*. Allen & Unwin, London.

Cornia, G.A. and Pannicia, R. (eds) (2000) *The Mortality Crisis in Transitional Economies*. Oxford University Press, Oxford.

Cornwell, J. (1984) *Hard-Earned Lives: Accounts of Health and Illness from East London*. Tavistock Publications, London and New York.

Coulter, A. (2001) 'Quality of hospital care: measuring patients' experiences', *Proceedings of the Royal College of Physicians of Edinburgh* 31: 34–6.

Coulter, A. (2002) *Ending Paternalism in Medical Care*, Nuffield Trust.

Coulter, A. *et al.* (1999) 'Sharing decisions with patients: is the information good enough?', *British Medical Journal* 318: 318–22.

Cox, C. and Mead, A. (eds) (1975) *A Sociology of Medical Practice*. Colller-Macmillan, London.

Craib. I. (1997) *Classical Social Theory*. Oxford University Press, Oxford.

Crick, B. (1982) *George Orwell: A Life*. Penguin, Harmondsworth.

Crompton, R. (1993) *Class and Stratification*. Polity Press.

Crow, G. and Allan, G. (1994) *Community Life: An introduction to local social relations*. Harvester Wheatsheaf.

Daily Telegraph (20.06.04) B. Brogran, 'One in two on disability claim for five years'.

Dalton, H. *et al.* (1997) 'Patent Threat to Research', *Nature* 385(6618): 672.

Davey-Smith, G., Dorling, D. and Shaw, M. (eds) (2001) *Poverty, Inequality and Health in Britain 1800–2000: A Reader*. The Policy Press, Bristol.

Davies, C. (1995) *Gender and the Professional Predicament in Nursing*. Open University Press, Buckingham.

Davis, F. (1960) 'Uncertainty in medical prognosis: clinical and functional', *American Journal of Sociology* 66: 41–7.

Department of Health (2000) *An Organisation with a Memory: report of an expert group on learning from adverse events in the NHS, Chaired by the Chief Medical Officer*. The Stationery Office, London.

Department of Health (2001) *The Expert Patient: A New Approach to Chronic Disease Management for the 21st Century*. Department of Health, London.

Department of Health (2002) *Learning from Bristol: The Department of Health's Response to the Report of the Public Inquiry into children's heart surgery at the Bristol Royal Infirmary 1984–1995*. Secretary of State for Health, London.

Department of Health (2003) *Health and Personal Social Services Statistics for England 2002–2003*. Department of Health, London.

Dickens, C. (1989) *Hard Times*. Oxford University Press, Oxford.

Dixon, A., Le Grand, J., Henderson, J., Murray, R. and Poteliakhoff (2003) 'Is the NHS equitable? a review of the evidence LSE Health and Social Care', *Discussion Paper No. 11*. London School of Economics.

Doran, T., Drever, F. and Whitehead (2004) 'Is there a north-south divide in social class inequalities in health in Great Britain? Cross sectional study using data from the 2001 census', *British Medical Journal* 328: 1043–5.

Dorling, D., Shaw, M. and Brimblecombe, N. (2000) 'Housing, wealth and community health: exploring the role of migration', in H. Graham (ed.) *Understanding Health Inequalities*. Open University Press, Buckingham.

Double, D. (2002) 'The limits of psychiatry', *British Medical Journal* 324: 900–4.

Durkheim, E. (1997) *The Division of Labor in Society*. The Free Press, New York.

Egolf, B., Lasker, J., Wolf, S., and Potvin, L. (1992) 'The Roseto effect: a 50-year comparison of mortality rates', *American Journal of Public Health* 82: 1089–92.

Elias, N. and Scotson, J.L. (1994) *The Established and the Outsiders: A Sociological Enquiry into Community Problems*. Sage Publications.

Elliman, D., Bedford, H. and Miller, E. (2001) 'MMR vaccine: Worries are not justified', *Archives of Disease in Childhood* 85: 271–4.

Elstad, J.I. (1998) 'The psycho-social perspective on social inequalities in health', in M. Bartley, D. Blane and G. Davey-Smith, *The Sociology of Health Inequalities*. Blackwell Publishers, Oxford.

Engels, F. (1969) *The Condition of the Working Class in England*. Panther Books.

Ferri, E. and Smith, K. (2003) 'Partnerships and parenthood', in Ferri, Bynner and Wadsworth.

Ferri, E., Bynner, J. and Wadsworth, M. (2003) *Changing Britain, Changing Lives: Three Generations at the Turn of the Century*. Institute of Education, University of London.

Ferrie, J.E., Shipley, M.J., Davey-Smith, G., Stansfeld, S.A. and Marmot, M.G. (2002) 'Change in health inequalities among British civil servants: the Whitehall II study', *Journal of Epidemiology and Community Health* 56: 922–6.

Ferris, P. (1967) *The Doctors*. Penguin, Harmondsworth.

Figlio, K. (1987) 'The lost subject of medical sociology', in G. Scambler (ed.) *Sociological Theory and Medical Sociology*. Tavistock Publications, London and New York.

Financial Times (14.04.04) R. Blutz, 'Anger at "lunatics" slur in voting guidelines'.

Financial Times (28.04.04) D. Firn and D. Turner 'Sick notes given a poor diagnosis'.

Finch, J. and Treanor, J. (2004) 'Boardroom pay bonanza goes on', *Guardian* 27.8.04.

Fitzpatrick, M. (1999) *The Tyranny of Health: doctors and the regulation of lifestyle*. Routledge, London.

Foster, P. (1995) *Women and the Health Care Industry: An Unhealthy Relationship?* Open University Press.

Frazer, W.M. (1950) *A History of English Public Health 1834–1939*. Baillière, Tindall and Cox, London.

Fremantle, N. and Hill, S. (2002) 'Medicalisation, limits to medicine, or never enough money to go round?', *British Medical Journal* 324: 864–5.

Freidson, E. (1960) 'Client Control and Medical Practice', *American Journal of Sociology* 65: 374–82.

Freidson, E. (1975) *The Profession of Medicine*. Dodd Mead, New York.

Gardner, K., Chapple, A. and Green, J. (1999) 'Barriers to referral in patients with angina: qualitative study', *British Medical Journal* 319: 418–21.

Gatrell, A. *et al.* (2002) 'Variations in use of tertiary cardiac services in part of North-West England', *Health and Place* 8 (3): 147–53.

General Medical Council (1998) 'Seeking patients' consent: the ethical considerations' November 1998.

Gerin, W., Pieper, C., Levy, R. and Pickering, T.G. (1992) 'Social support in social interactions: A moderator of cardiovascular reactivity', *Psychosomatic Medicine* 54: 324–36.

Geronimus, A. *et al.* (1996) 'Excess mortality among blacks and whites in the United States', *New England Journal of Medicine* 335: 1552–8.

Goddard, M. and Smith, P. (2001) 'Equity of access to health care services', *Social Science and Medicine* 53 (9): 1149–62.

Goffman, E. (1968) *Stigma: Notes on the Management of Spoiled Identity.* Penguin, Harmondsworth.

Goldman, L. and Cook, E.F. (1984) 'The decline in ischemic heart disease mortality rates: an analysis of the comparative effects of medical interventions and changes in lifestyle', *Annals of Internal Medicine* 101: 825–36.

Goldstein, R. (1991) 'The Implicated and the Immune: responses to AIDS in the Arts and Popular Culture' in D. Nelkin, D.P. Willis and V.S. Parris, *A Disease of Society: Cultural and Institutional Responses to AIDS.* Cambridge University Press, Cambridge.

Graham, H. (1990) 'Behaving Well: Women's health behaviour in context', in H. Roberts (ed.) *Women's Health Counts.* Routledge, London and New York.

Graham, H. (ed.) (2000) *Understanding Health Inequalities.* Open University Press, Buckingham.

Graham, H. and Oakley, A. (1986) 'Competing Ideologies of Reproduction: Medical and Maternal Perspectives on Pregnancy', in H. Roberts (ed.) *Women, Health and Reproduction.* Routledge & Kegan Paul, London.

Gray, P. (1999) *Mental Health in the Workplace: tackling the effects of stress.* The Mental Health Foundation, London.

Grayling, A.C. (2003) *What is Good?: The Search for the Best Way to Live.* Phoenix.

Guardian (10.11.98) D. Ward, 'Three seek right to sex change operation funded by the NHS'.

Guardian (22.12.98) J. Welson, 'Sex-change trio win NHS test case'.

Guardian (30.07.99) C. Dyer, 'Ban on operation for sex change was unlawful'.

Guardian (01.02.2000) G. Seenan 'Healthy limbs cut off at patients' request'.

Guardian (01.04.04) C. Denny, 'Labour to tackle inner-city "culture of worklessness"'.

Guardian (15.04.04) J. Meikle, 'A friend can mend a broken heart'.

Guardian (03.07.04) J. Carvel, 'Patients to be customers in new NHS'.

Guardian (03.08.04) R. James, 'Cut it out, please'.

Guardian (25.08.04) E. Peck, 'Force for Good Society'.

Guardian (08.09.04) J. Moorhead, 'The home birth lottery'.

Guardian (18.09.04) M. Jacques, 'The death of intimacy'.

Guardian (18.11.04) J. Meikle, 'Gulf war syndrome is genuine says law lords enquiry'.

Guardian (03.12.04) S. Bowers, 'GPs worry over sick note "spies" in the surgery'.

Halsey, A.H. (ed.) (1988) *British Social Trends Since 1900.* Macmillan, London.

Hammond, R. and Rowell, A. (2001) 'Trust Us: We're the Tobacco Industry'. Campaign for Tobacco-Free Kids (US) and Action on Smoking and Health (UK). Available online at www.ash.org.uk.

Handy, C. (1998) *The Hungry Spirit.* Arrow Books, London.

Harding, R., Sherr, L., Sherr, A., Moorhead, R. and Singh, S. (2003) 'Welfare rights advice in primary care: prevalence, processes and specialist provision', *Family Practice* 20 (1): 48–53.

Hart, J.T. (1971) 'The inverse care law', *The Lancet*, 27 February.

Hart J.T. (1975) 'Clinical and economic consequences of patients as producers', *Journal of Public Health Medicine* 17: 383–6.

Hart, J.T. (1998) 'Viewpoint: expectations of health care: promoted, managed or shared?', *Health Expectations* 1 (1): 3–13.

Hart, A. and Lockey, R. (2002) 'Inequalities in health care provision: the relationship between contemporary health policy and contemporary practice in maternity services in England', *Journal of Advanced Nursing* 37 (5): 485–93.

Hart, G. and Wellings, K. (2002) 'Sexual behaviour and its medicalisation: in sickness and in health', *British Medical Journal* 324: 896–900.

Hattersley, L. (1999) 'Trends in life expectancy by social class – an update' *Health Statistics Quarterly* 2: 16–24.

Haywood, S. and Alaszewski, A. (1980) *Crisis in the Health Service*. Croom Helm, London.

Healy, D. (2004) 'Hey, this new drug – it's to die for . . .', *Times Higher* 10.9.04.

Hillier, S. (1987) 'Rationalism, bureaucracy, and the organization of the health services: Max Weber's contribution to understanding modern health care systems', in G. Scambler (ed.) *Health and Social Change: A Critical Theory*. Open University Press.

Hirschman, Albert O. (1970) *Exit, Voice, and Loyalty: Responses to Decline in Firms, Organizations, and States*. Harvard University Press.

HM Treasury/Department of Health (2002) *Cross Cutting Review: Tackling Health Inequalities*. Department of Health, London.

Hochschild, A. (1983) *The Managed Heart: Commercialization of Human Feeling*. University of California Press.

Hoskins, R. and Carter, D.E. (2000) 'Welfare benefits' screening and referral: a new direction for community nurses?' *Health and Social Care in the Community* 8 (6): 390–7.

Hoskins, R.A.J. and Smith, L.N. (2002) 'Nurse-led welfare benefits screening in a General Practice located in a deprived area', *Public Health* 116 (4): 214–20.

Hunt, T. (2004) *Building Jerusalem: The Rise and Fall of the Victorian City*. Weidenfeld & Nicolson, London

Illich, I. (1977) *Limits to Medicine: Medical Nemesis: The Expropriation of Health*. Penguin, Harmondsworth.

James, N. (1989) 'Emotional Labour, skills and work in the social regulation of feeling', *The Sociological Review* 37 (1): 15–42.

James, N. (1992) 'Care = organisation + physical labour + emotional labour', *Sociology of Health and Illness* 14: 488–509.

Jewson, N. (1976) 'The disappearance of the sick-man from medical cosmologies: 1770–1870', *Sociology* 10: 225.

Jobling, R. (1988) 'The Experience of Psoriasis Under Treatment', in R. Anderson and M. Bury *Living with Chronic Illness: The Experiences of Patients and their Families*. Unwin Hyman, London.

Judge, K. (1995) 'Income distribution and life expectancy: a critical appraisal', *British Medical Journal* 311: 1282–5.

Kelleher, D. (1994) 'Self-help groups and their relationship to medicine', in J. Gabe, D. Kelleher and G. Williams, *Challenging Medicine*. Routledge, London.

Kennedy, A.D.M. *et al.* (2002) 'Effects of decision aids for menorrhagia on treatment choices, health outcomes, and costs', *Journal of the American Medical Association* 288: 21.

Kennedy, I. (1981) *The Unmasking of Medicine: The 1980 Reith Lectures*. George Allen & Unwin, London.

Kennedy, I. (2001) *Learning from Bristol: The report of the public inquiry into children's heart surgery at the Bristol Royal Infirmary 1984–1995*. Secretary of State for Health.

Kivimaki, M. *et al.* (2002) 'Work stress and risk of cardiovascular mortality: prospective cohort study of industrial employees' *British Medical Journal* 325.

Klein, R. (1989) *The Politics of the National Health Service* (2nd edn). Longman, London and New York.

Koos E.L. (1954) *The Health of Regionville*. Columbia University Press, New York.

Kouzis, A.C. and Eaton, W.W. (1998) 'Absence of social networks, social support and health services utilization', *Psychological Medicine* 28: 1301–10.

Kralik, D., Brown, M. and Koch, T. (2001) 'Women's experience of "being diagnosed" with a long-term illness', *Journal of Advanced Nursing* 33 (5): 594–602.

Laird, S. (2004) *First Contact*, MedEconomics, September.

Lantz, P.M. *et al.* (1998) 'Socio-economic factors, health behaviours and mortality', *Journal of the American Medical Association* 279 (21): 1703–8.

Le Grand, J. and Dixon, A. (2004) *Patient Choice and Equity in the National Health Service.* London School of Economics.

Lee, D. and Newby, H. (1983) *The Problem of Sociology: An introduction to the discipline.* Unwin Hyman, London.

Lee, E., Clements, S., Ingham, R. and Stone, N. (2004) *A Matter of Choice? Explaining national variations in teenage abortion and motherhood.* Joseph Rowntree Foundation.

Lipsky, M. (1980) *Street Level Bureaucrats: Dilemmas of the individual in public services.* Russell Sage, New York.

Littler, C. (1982) *The Development of the Labour Process in Capitalist Societies: a Comparative Analysis of Work Organisation in Britain, the USA, and Japan.* Heinemann, London.

Loumidis, J., Youngs, R., Lessof, C. and Stafford, B. (2001) *New Deal for Disabled People: National Survey of Incapacity Benefits Claimants.* DWP Research Report 160.

Lukes, S. (1974) *Power: A Radical View.* Macmillan, London.

Lukes, S. (1992) *Emile Durkheim: His life and works, a historical and critical study.* Penguin, Harmondsworth.

Lynch, J. *et al.* (1997) 'Workplace conditions socioeconomic status and the risk of mortality and acute myocardial infarction: the Kuopio ischemic heart disease risk factor study', *American Journal of Public Health* 87: 617–22.

Mackenbach, J.P., Bouvier-Colle, M.H. and Jougla, E. (1990) ' "Avoidable" mortality and health services: a review of aggregate data studies', *Journal of Epidemiology and Community Health* 44: 106–11.

Macpherson, Sir William (1999) *The Stephen Lawrence Inquiry Report.* Secretary of State for the Home Department, London.

Magnet, J. (2003) 'What's wrong with nursing?', *Prospect*, December 2003.

Manpower (2000) Press Release: Irish holiday entitlements lowest in Europe. 17 December. Manpower, Dublin.

Marmot, M. (2004) *Status Syndrome: How Your Social Standing Directly Affects Your Health and Life Expectancy.* Bloomsbury, London.

Marshall, T.H. (1950) 'Citizenship and Social Class', in T.H. Marshall and T. Bottomore (1992) *Citizenship and Social Class.* Pluto Press, London.

Martin J.P. (1984) *Hospitals in Trouble.* Blackwell.

Marx, K. (1974) *Economic and Philosophical Manuscripts of 1844.* Lawrence and Wishart, London.

Marx, K. (1976) *Capital, Vol 1.* Penguin, Harmondsworth.

Marx, K. (1978) *The Eighteenth Brumaire of Louis Bonaparte.* Foreign Languages Press, Peking.

McAlister, F.A. *et al.* (2004) 'Influence of socioeconomic deprivation on the primary care burden and treatment of patients with a diagnosis of heart failure in general practice in Scotland: population based study', *British Medical Journal*, 23 April.

McClure, R.J., Newell, S.J. and Edwards, S. (1996) 'Patient characteristics affecting attendance at general outpatient clinics', *Archives of Disease in Childhood* 74 (2): 121–5.

McCormick, A., Fleming, D. and Charlton, J. (1995) 'Which patients consult: a multivariate analysis of socio-economic factors', in *Morbidity Statistics from General Practice:*

Fourth National Study 1991–1992. Office of Population Censuses and Surveys, HMSO, London.

McKeown, T. (1976) *The Modern Rise of Population*. Edward Arnold, London.

McKeown, T. (1979) *The Role of Medicine: Dream, Mirage or Nemesis?* Basil Blackwell, Oxford.

Mills, C.W. (2000) *The Sociological Imagination: Fortieth Anniversary edition*. Oxford University Press, Oxford.

Mintzes, B. (2002) 'Direct to consumer advertising is medicalizing normal human experience: For', *British Medical Journal* 324: 908–9.

Modell, B. *et al.* (2000) 'Informed choice in genetic screening for thalassaemia during pregnancy: audit from a national confidential inquiry', *British Medical Journal* 320: 337–41.

Monbiot, G. (2001) *Captive State: The Corporate Takeover of Britain*. Pan Books, London.

MORI Social Research Institute (2003) *Exploring Trust in Public Institutions*. MORI Social Research Institute.

Morris, J. and Titmuss, R. (1944) 'Epidemiology of peptic ulcer: vital statistics', *The Lancet* ii: 841–5.

Moynihan, R. (2003) 'The making of a disease: female sexual dysfunction', *British Medical Journal* 326: 45–7.

Moynihan, R., Heath, I. and Henry, D. (2002) 'Selling sickness: the pharmaceutical industry and disease mongering', *British Medical Journal* 324: 886–91.

Mulcahy, L. (2003) *Disputing Doctors: the socio-dynamics of complaints about medical care*. Open University Press, Buckingham.

Mullen, K. (1992) 'A question of balance: health behaviour and work context among male Glaswegians' *Sociology of Health and Illness* 14 (1): 72–97.

National Institute for Clinical Excellence (2004a) 'Depression: Management of depression in primary and secondary care' *Clinical Guideline 23*. NICE, London.

National Institute for Clinical Excellence (2004b) 'Caesarian Section', *Clinical Guideline 13*. Developed by the National Collaborating Centre for Women's and Children's Health. NICE, London.

O'Brien, M. (1994) 'The managed heart revisited: health and social control', *The Sociological Review* 42 (3): 393–413.

O'Cathain, A. *et al.* (2002) 'Use of evidence based leaflets to promote informed choice in maternity care: randomised control trial in everyday practice', *British Medical Journal* 324: 643–6.

O'Conner, A.M. *et al.* (1999) 'Decision aids for patients facing health treatment or screening decisions: systematic review', *British Medical Journal* 319: 731–43.

Office of National Statistics (2004) *The National Statistics Socio-Economic Classification User Manual*. Office for National Statistics, London.

Oliver, A. *et al.* (2002) 'Addressing Health Inequalities', *The Lancet* 306: 565–7.

Open University (1985) *Caring for Health: Dilemmas and Prospects*, Course book for course U205: Health and Disease. Open University Press, Milton Keynes.

Opie, A. (1997) 'Thinking teams and thinking clients: issues of discourse and representation in the work of health teams', *Sociology of Health and Illness* 19 (3): 259–80.

Orwell, S. and Angus, I. (1970) *The Collected Essays, Journalism and Letters of George Orwell, Volume 4*. Penguin Books.

Owens, P. and Glennester, H. (1990) *Nursing in Conflict*. Macmillan, London.

Pahl, J. (ed.) (1985) *Private Violence and Public Policy: The Needs of Battered Women and the Responses of the Public Services*. Routledge & Kegan Paul.

Palmer, T., Granger, H. and Fitzner, G. (2004) *Trade Union Membership 2003*. Department of Trade and Industry, London.

Parkin, F. (2002) *Max Weber*. Routledge, London.

Payne, N. and Saul, C. (1997) 'Variations in the use of cardiology services in a health authority: comparison of coronary artery revascularisation rates with prevalence of angina and coronary mortality', *British Medical Journal* 314: 257.

Perkin, H. (1989) *The Rise of Professional Society: England Since 1880*. Routledge, London and New York.

Phillips, Lord of Worth Matravers (2000) *The BSE Inquiry: The inquiry into BSE and Variant CJD in the United Kingdom*. HMSO, London.

Piachaud, D. (1993) 'Poverty in the United Kingdom', in P. Townsend, *The International Analysis of Poverty*. Harvester Wheatsheaf.

Pilgrim, D. and Rogers, A. (1993) *A Sociology of Mental Health and Illness*. Open University Press.

Pollitt, C. (1987) 'Performance measurement and the consumer: hijacking the bandwagon?' in *Performance Measurement and the Consumer*. National Consumer Council, London.

Pollock, A. (2004) *NHS plc: The Privatisation of our Health Care*. Verso.

Porter, R. (1999) *The Greatest Benefit to Mankind: A Medical History of Humanity from Antiquity to the Present*. Fontana Press, London.

Porter, R. (2000) *Enlightenment: Britain and the Creation of the Modern World*. Penguin Books.

Prior, L. (2003) 'Belief, knowledge, and expertise: the emergence of the lay expert in medical sociology', *Sociology of Health and Illness* 25: 41–57.

Putnam, R. (2000) *Bowling Alone: The Collapse and Revival of American Community*. Simon & Schuster.

Raleigh, V.S. and Clifford, G.M. (2002) 'Knowledge, perceptions and care of people with diabetes in England and Wales', *Journal of Diabetes Nursing* 6 (3): 72–8.

Redfern, M. (2001) *The Royal Liverpool Children's Inquiry Report*. House of Commons, London.

Richards, H.M., Reid, M.E. and Watt, G.C.M. (2002) 'Socioeconomic variations in responses to chest pain: qualitative study', *British Medical Journal* 324: 1308.

Rowntree, B.S. (1941) *Poverty and Progress*. Longman, London.

Runciman, W.G. (1972) *Relative Deprivation and Social Justice: a study of attitudes to social inequality in twentieth-century England*. Penguin, Harmondsworth.

Russell, B. (1976) *In Praise of Idleness and Other Essays*. George Allen & Unwin, London.

Salmon, J.W. (1984) 'Organizing medical care for profit', in J.B. McKinlay (ed.) *Issues in the Political Economy of Health Care*. Tavistock Publications.

Sanders, D. and Carver, R. (1985) *The Struggle for Health: Medicine and the Politics of Underdevelopment*. Macmillan.

Salvage, J. (2002) *Rethinking Professionalism: the first step for patient-focused care?* Institute for Public Policy Research Future Health Worker Project.

Scambler, G. (2002) *Health and Social Change: A critical theory*. Open University Press, Buckingham.

Scheff, T. (1963) 'Decision rules, types of error, and their consequences' in D. Tuckett and J.M. Kaufert (eds) (1978) *Basic Readings in Medical Sociology*. Tavistock Publications.

Secretary of State for Health (2000) *The NHS Plan: a plan for investment, a plan for reform*. Department of Health, London.

Secretary of State for Health (2004) Speech by Rt Hon John Reid MP, Secretary of State for Health, to the Chief Executives Conference, 3 February. Department of Health, London.

Sefton, T. (2002) 'Recent Changes in the Distribution of the Social Wage' CASE paper 62. Centre for Analysis of Social Exclusion, London School of Economics, London.

Sennett, R. (1998) *The Corrosion of Character: The Personal Consequences of Work in the New Capitalism*. Norton, New York.

Sheaff, M. (1997) 'Urban Partnerships, Economic Regeneration and the "Healthy City"', in N. Jewson and S. MacGregor, *Transforming Cities: Contested Governance and New Spatial Divisions*. Routledge, London and New York.

Sheaff, M. (2003) Inequalities in health services and the 'inverse care law', Paper presented to the World Health Organisation International Healthy Cities Conference, Belfast October.

Simpson, K. (1985) 'Authority and responsibility delegation predicts quality of care', *Journal of Advanced Nursing* 10: 345–8.

Smith, A. (1804) 'An inquiry into the nature and causes of the wealth of nations'. Cited in Davey-Smith, Dorling and Shaw (2001).

Smith, P. (1991) 'The nursing process: raising the profile of emotional care in nurse training', *Journal of Advanced Nursing* 16: 74–81.

South East Regional Office, NHS Executive (2000) *Managed Clinical Networks*. Department of Health.

Spiegel, D., Bloom, J., Kraemer, H. and Gottheil, E. (1989) 'The beneficial effect of psychosocial treatment on survival of metastatic breast cancer patients: A randomized prospective outcome study', *The Lancet* 12: 888–91.

Stacey, M. (1992) *Regulating British Medicine: the General Medical Council*. Wiley, Chichester.

Stacey, M. (1976) 'The health service consumer: a sociological misconception', *Sociological Review Monograph 22, The Sociology of the NHS*. Blackwell.

Stacey, M., Dearden, R., Pill, R. and Robinson, D. (1970) *Hospitals, Children and their Families: The Report of a Pilot Study*. Routledge & Kegan Paul, London.

Stansfield, S.A., Fuhrer, R. and Shipley, M.J. (1998) 'Types of social support as predictors of psychiatric morbidity in a cohort of British Civil Servants (Whitehall II Study) (Support and Psychiatric Morbidity)', *Psychological Medicine* 28: 881–92.

Stedman Jones, G. (2004) *An End to Poverty: A Historical Debate*. Profile Books, London.

Stirling, A.M., Wilson, P. and McConnachie, A. (2001) 'Deprivation, psychological stress and consultation length in general practice', *British Journal of General Practice 2001* 51 (467): 456–60.

Strauss, A., Fagerhaugh S., Suczek B. and Wiener C. (1982) 'Sentimental work in the technologized hospital', *Sociology of Health and Illness* 4 (3): 254–78.

Sunday Telegraph (20.06.04) E. Day, 'Unhappy with their life, work and love – that's Britain's 30-year-olds'.

Surowiecki, J. (2004) *The Wisdom of Crowds: Why the Many are Smarter than the Few*. Little, Brown.

Sutherland, Prof. Sir Stewart (1999) 'With Respect to Old Age: Long Term Care – Rights and Responsibilities' A Report by the Royal Commission on Long Term Care Chairman, Prof. Sir Stewart Sutherland. The Stationery Office.

Szreter, S. (2001) 'The importance of social intervention in Britain's mortality decline c. 1850–1914: a re-interpretation of the role of public health', in B. Davey, A. Gray and C. Seale *Health and Disease: A Reader* (3rd edition) Open University Press.

Sztompka, P. (1999) *Trust: A Sociological Theory*. Cambridge University Press, Cambridge.

Tawney, R.H. (1952) *Equality*. Allen & Unwin, London.

Taylor, C. (1991) *The Ethics of Authenticity*. Harvard University Press.

Taylor, F.W. (1911) *The Principles of Scientific Management*. Harper, New York.

The Independent (21.09.04) R. Horton, 'Obstacles to Truth'.

The Observer (22.02.04) J. Fineman, 'Maverick view that sparked panic over the triple vaccine'.

The Observer (29.09.04) C. Barron, 'Big Pharma shared by net'.

The Scottish Office (1998) *Acute Services Review Report*. Department of Health.

Thompson, E.P. (1980) *The Making of the English Working Class*. Penguin, Harmondsworth.

Thompson, K. and Tunstall, J. (eds) (1971) *Sociological Perspectives: Selected Readings*. Penguin, Harmondsworth.

Titmuss, R.M. (1968) 'Commitment to Welfare', in E. Butterworth and D. Weir (eds) (1976) *The Sociology of Modern Britain*. Fontana/Collins.

Tod, A.M., Read, C., Lacey, A. and Abbott, J. (2001) 'Barriers to uptake of services for coronary heart disease: qualitative study', *British Medical Journal* 323: 214.

Townsend, P. (1974) 'Poverty as relative deprivation: resources and style of living', in D. Wedderburn, *Poverty, Inequality and Class Structure*. Cambridge University Press, Cambridge.

Townsend, P. (1979) *Poverty in the United Kingdom: A survey of household resources and standards of living*. Penguin, Harmondsworth.

Townsend, P. and Davidson, N. (1982) *Inequalities in Health: The Black Report*. Penguin, Harmondsworth.

TUC (2004) *Defending Incapacity Benefit*. Trades Union Congress, October 2004.

Tuckett, D. and Kaufert, J.M. (eds) (1978) *Basic Readings in Medical Sociology*. Tavistock Publications.

Uchino, B.N. (1999) *Social Support, Physiological Processes and Health, Current Directions in Psychological Science*. American Psychology Association.

United Nations (1995) *Report of the World Summit for Social Development* (Copenhagen 6–12 March). United Nations, New York.

Van Bastelaer, A. and Vaguer, C. (2004) *Working Times: Statistics in Focus: Population and Social Conditions*. Eurostat, Luxembourg.

Waitzkin, H. (1991) *The Politics of Medical Encounters: How Patients and Doctors Deal with Social Problems*. Yale University Press, New Haven and London.

Wakefield, A. *et al.* (1998) 'Ileal-lymphoid-nodular hyperplasia, non-specific colitis and pervasive developmental disorder in children', *The Lancet* 351: 9103.

Walberg, P., McKee, M., Shkolnikov, V., Chenet, L. and Leon, D.A. (1998) 'Economic change, crime and mortality crisis in Russia: regional analysis', *British Medical Journal* 317: 312–18.

Walby, S. *et al.* (1994) *Medicine and Nursing: Professions in a Changing Health Service*. Sage Publications.

Weber, M. (1930) *The Protestant Ethic and the Spirit of Capitalism*. Allen & Unwin, London.

Weber, M. (1948) From *Max Weber: Essays in Sociology*, edited by H. Gerth and C.W. Mills. Routledge & Kegan Paul, London.

Weber, M. (1952) *Ancient Judaism*. Free Press, Glencoe.

Weber, M. (1968) *Economy and Society – an outline of interpretive sociology*, trans. G. Roth and G. Wittich. Bedminster Press, New York.

Webster, C. (1986) 'The origins of social medicine in Britain', *Bulletin of the Society for the Social History of Medicine* 38: 52–5.

Webster, C. (ed.) (1991) *Aneurin Bevan on the National Health Service*. University of Oxford Wellcome Unit for the History of Medicine, Oxford.

Weich, S., Lewis, G. and Jenkins, S.P. (2002) 'Income inequality and self-rated health in Britain', *Journal of Epidemiology and Community Health* 56 (6) 436–441.

Wheen, F. (1999) *Karl Marx*. Fourth Estate, London.

White, L. and Cant, B. (2003) 'Social networks, social support, health and HIV-positive gay men' *Health and Social Care in the Community* 11 (4): 329–34.

Whitehead, M. (1992) 'The Health Divide', in P. Townsend, N. Davidson and M. Whitehead *Inequalities in Health: The Black Report and the Health Divide*. Penguin, Harmondsworth.

Whitehead, M. *et al.* (1997) 'As the health divide widens in Sweden and Britain, what's happening to access to care?' *British Medical Journal* 315: 1006–9.

Wilkinson, R. (1996) *Unhealthy Societies: The Afflictions of Inequality*. Routledge.

Willetts, D. (1992) *Modern Conservatism*. Penguin, Harmondsworth.

Willetts, D. (1997) *Why Vote Conservative?* Penguin, Harmondsworth.

Williams, R. (1983) 'Concepts of Health: An Analysis of Lay Logic', *Sociology* 17 (2): 185–205.

Williams, S. (1987) 'Goffman, interactionism, and the management of stigma in everyday life', in G. Scambler (ed.) *Sociological Theory and Medical Sociology*. Tavistock Publications.

Wittenberg, R., Comas-Herrera, A., Pickard, L. and Hancock, C. (2004) *Future demand for long-term care in the UK*. Joseph Rowntree Foundation/London School of Economics.

Wolff, J. (2002) *Why Read Marx Today*. Oxford University Press, Oxford.

World Health Organization (2000) *World Health Report 2000 – Health Systems: Improving Performance*. WHO, Geneva.

Wuthnow, R. (1998) *Loose Connections: Joining Together in America's Fragmented Communities*. Harvard University Press, Cambridge, MA.

Young, M. and Willmott, P. (1957) *Family and Kinship in East London*. Routledge & Kegan Paul, London.

Zeitlin, I.M. (1968) *Ideology and the Development of Sociological Theory*. Prentice Hall, Englewood Cliffs, NJ.

Zola, I.K. (1972) 'Medicine as an Institution of Social Control' in C. Cox and A. Mead (eds) (1975) *A Sociology of Medical Practice*. Collier-Macmillan, London.

Zola, I.K. (1975) 'Culture and symptoms: an analysis of patients' presenting complaints', in C. Cox and A. Mead, *A Sociology of Medical Practice*. Collier-Macmillan, London.

Index

The index is in word-by-word order. Page numbers in *italics* refer to tables and diagrams.

SOCIAL POLICY

An Introduction

Second Edition

Ken Blakemore

Praise for the first edition:
  "Clear, concise, up-to-date and helpfully referenced"
      Professor Ian Kendall, University of Portsmouth, SPA News.

Praise for the second edition:
  "A substantial introductory text. Excellent inclusion of employment policy, health / social care/ housing and environment."
      Sheila Emmett, Sunderland University

This edition of *Social Policy: An Introduction* builds on the strengths of the
highly respected first edition to offer a broad introduction to current developments in social policy and welfare. Comprehensive, readable and thought-
provoking, this is now the standard introductory book on social policy in the
United Kingdom.

The completely revised second edition has been expanded and updated to
reflect latest developments in the major fields of social welfare;

- New chapters on employment policy and on the impact of devolution and
  the European Union
- Completely re-written chapters on social security and poverty, education,
  health, housing and environment, social care, and the history and principles
  of social policy
- Discussion and analysis of major policy themes including power and decision-making, paying for welfare, social control and the role of the professions
- Study aids include glossary of key terms; each chapter includes key terms
  and concepts and further reading

Social Policy: An Introduction is essential reading for students beginning or
building on their study of social policy or welfare. It can be used in under-
graduate degree courses, postgraduate diplomas and Masters level, A-level,
HND, HNC Certificate and Diploma studies. The book is an invaluable
reference resource for practitioners, professionals of policy makers in fields
including health, medicine and nursing, housing, social services and counselling, education, law and criminology.

Contents: *The author - Preface - Acknowledgements - The subject of social policy
- Ideas and concepts in social policy - The development of social policy in Britain -
Who gets what? Slicing the welfare cake - Social policy, politics and social control -
Who makes social policy? The example of education - Work and welfare - Are
professionals good for you? The example of health policy and health professionals -
Utopias and ideals: Housing policy and the environment - Community and social
care - Devolution and social policy - Conclusion: The future of social policy -
Glossary - Bibliography - Index.*

320pp 0 335 20847 9 (Paperback)

THINKING NURSING

Tom Mason and Elizabeth Whitehead

This major new textbook provides a unique one-stop resource that introduces nursing students to the disciplines that underpin nursing practice. The broad range of subjects covered includes Sociology, Psychology, Anthropology, Public Health, Philosophy, Economics, Politics and Science.

Written by nursing lecturers with nursing students in mind, this book enables nurses to grasp the principles behind these disciplines and apply the concepts to everyday health care practices. Each chapter offers:

- The theoretical background of the major tenets of each discipline
- A comprehensive discussion of how they relate to practice
- Cross-references to other relevant chapter sections
- Suggestions for further reading
- A glossary of key terms.

Practical advice is also available in a chapter dedicated to methods of research, planning and construction of written work. Moreover, the textbook is designed to encourage creative and lateral thinking beyond its use in planning and writing assignments.

Thinking Nursing is essential reading for nursing students on Common Foundation Programmes (both at diploma and degree level) and qualified nurses undertaking additional specialist training including masters degrees, as well as those involved in planning, designing and the implementation of educational courses for nurses.

Contents: *Introduction – Thinking Sociology – Thinking Psychology – Thinking Anthropology – Thinking Public Health – Thinking Philosophy – Thinking Economics – Thinking Politics – Thinking Science – Thinking Writing – Conclusions – References – Index.*

456pp 0 335 21040 6 (Paperback) 0 335 21041 4 (Hardback)

A SOCIOLOGY OF MENTAL HEALTH AND ILLNESS
Third Edition

Anne Rogers and David Pilgrim

- How have sociologists theorized and researched mental health and illness?
- In what ways do sociologists approach this topic differently to those from other disciplines?
- How do we understand mental health problems in their social context?

This bestselling book provides a clear overview of the major aspects of the sociology of mental health and illness, and helps students to develop a critical approach to the subject. In this new edition, the authors update each of the chapters, taking into consideration recent relevant literature from social science and social psychiatry. A new chapter has been included on the impact of stigma, which covers an analysis of the responses of the lay public to mental health and illness and representations of mental health (particularly in the media) in a post-institutional context.

A Sociology of Mental Health and Illness is a key teaching and learning resource for undergraduates and postgraduates studying a range of medical sociology and health related courses, as well as trainee mental health workers in the fields of social work, nursing, clinical psychology and psychiatry.

Contents: *Acknowledgements – Introduction – Perspectives on mental health and illness – Stigma re-visited and lay representations of mental health problems – Social class and mental health – Women and men – Race and ethnicity – Age and ageing – The mental health professions – The treatment of people with mental health problems – The organization of mental health work – Psychiatry and legal control – Users of mental health services – References – Index.*

272pp 0 35 21583 1 (Paperback) 0 335 21584 X (Hardback)

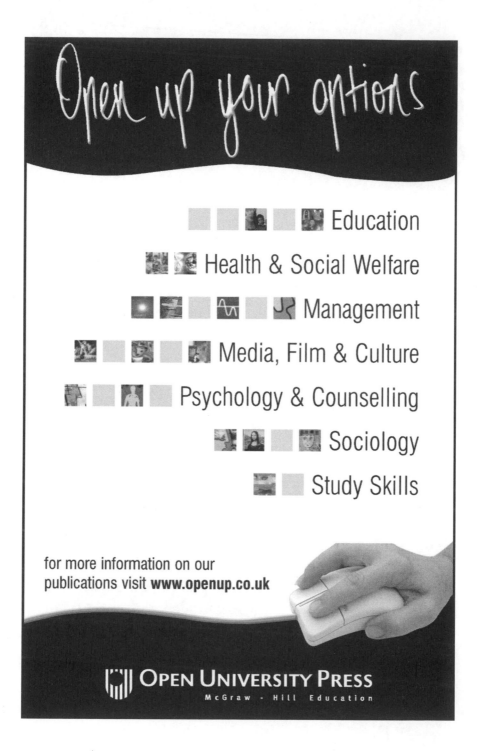